Charles de Mertens

An Account of the Plague
Which Raged at Moscow, 1771

LONDON, 1799

With a long introduction, and annotated
bibliography by Professor John Alexander,
University of Kansas, Lawrence.

ORIENTAL RESEARCH PARTNERS
NEWTONVILLE, MASS.
1977

ISBN 0-89250-007-7

Note on this volume

Eighteenth century printers at times falsely numbered the pages to make their books appear larger than was the case. This book is one such sample with page 65 following page 48. The text remains intact.

A catalogue outlining our other books
in the Russian history field will be sent upon
request. Please write to the Editor,
Dr. P.H. Clendenning, Oriental Research Partners,
Box 158, Newtonville, Mass. 02160.

INTRODUCTORY NOTE

British Responses to the Moscow Plague of 1771

The English translation of Charles de Mertens' account of the plague
epidemic in Russia in 1770-72 sprang from an earlier and larger phenomenon:
British apprehension about, and responses to, the most spectacular European
epidemic since the pestilence at Marseilles fifty years earlier. Just as
wars invariably evoke literary refighting of the contest among the partici-
pants and their partisans, so major epidemics often engender comment and
controversy. Charles de Mertens became embroiled in just such a medico-
historical debate. First published in Latin in 1778, his book apprised the
European reading public of the beginnings of a debate about the plague in
Russia. Its popularity and translation into German (1779), French (1784),
Italian (1786), and English (1799) mirrored European interest in the subject
and also stimulated other eyewitnesses to publish their recollections of
the epidemic and their thoughts about plague in general.

From a wider perspective, the medical disputes over the Moscow epidemic
represented a revival and an extension to Russia of earlier European debates
about the nature of plague. The Russia-oriented phase of this debate continued into the first decades of the nineteenth century when, like the
plague itself, it lapsed for nearly fifty years. Controversy resumed upon
the occasion of the plague outbreak of 1877-78 on the lower Volga, and it
persisted through the discovery of the plague bacillus in Hong Kong in 1894
and the establishment of the rat-flea nexus during the next decade. In the
conquest of epidemic plague, then, Mertens' book forms one link in a chain of
medical theorizing and historical observation that extends back to the time
of Hippocrates. If that seems faint praise, one should remember that modern
epidemiology stands on a long progression of past achievement, and that
Mertens' account provoked extensive discussion and provided an insightful,

widely read account of the last major outbreak of plague on European soil.
Thus his book deserves republication as an important source for both Russian
and general medical history and, not least, as a vivid and perceptive description of a spectacular instance of epidemic disease in a major European
city.

To understand the lively reception that Mertens' contemporaries gave
his book, one must examine earlier European reactions to the epidemic. The
plague of 1770-72 in Russia stimulated intense interest abroad because it
burst upon a political situation already charged with danger to the peace
of Europe. Civil war in the moribund Polish-Lithuanian Commonwealth, aggravated by mounting Russian political and military intervention, had led
to war between Russia and the Ottoman Empire in the fall of 1768. Dazzling
Russian victories on land and sea--the invasion and occupation of the
Danubian Principalities in 1769-70, the destruction of the Turkish fleet
at Chesme in 1771, and the conquest of the Crimea in 1771--threatened to
deform the European balance of power by amputating its ailing southeastern
appendages, Poland and Turkey. Prussia, Russia's ally since 1764, and
Austria both claimed compensation for Russia's growing power in eastern
and southern Europe, acting on Empress Catherine II's own later dictum that,
in international politics "he who gets nothing, loses." As Russia alone
could not suppress the Poles and defeat the Turks simultaneously, Austria
and Prussia exploited the situation to seize territory along their fron-
tiers with Poland. The first partition of Poland, agreed upon in 1772 and
promulgated in 1773, resulted.[1]

At the same time other nations of Europe stirred with tension: Sweden
from the rivalries of crown, estates, and foreign powers that, unlike those
in Poland, spawned a royal coup d'etat in 1772; Denmark from the turbulent

reform ministry of Struensee, in 1770-71; Britain from parliamentary turmoil,
competition with France and Spain, and rumblings in her North American
colonies; France from her efforts to counter Russian influence in Sweden,
Poland, and Turkey, and from Maupeou's struggle against the parlements.[2]
In 1770, then, European nerves were taut and much attention focused on developments in the southeast. Small wonder that the sudden intrusion of pestilence
into that region touched off consternation throughout Europe.

More fearsome than any immediate political impact of the plague was
the possibility of its following the trade routes to northern and western
Europe, which had been free from the disease since the early decades of the
century. Poland, Austria, Prussia, Sweden, and Russia all instituted cordons
and quarantines against the pestilential peril.[3] Great Britain's extensive
trade through the Baltic, her growing commerce with the Mediterranean, and
popular remembrance of earlier epidemics, especially the London plague of
1665, caused the royal government and its representatives abroad to appraise
the threat and to undertake precautions. Meanwhile the British and conti-
nental press snatched at every mention of pestilence. Though the plague
scare blew over by the end of 1772, it left Europeans with a sharpened
awareness of their ignorance and helplessness in the face of the mysterious
malady that still lurked in the southeast.

In the years after the epidemic, before European apprehensions had re-
ceded, Mertens and other medical writers sought to dispel popular fears by
explaining what had happened in Moscow in 1770-72 and by suggesting how the
tragedy might have been averted. Most of these writers took an activist
approach to the disease; they believed it could be prevented or at least
limited. Some speculated about using inoculations to thwart pestilence,
reasoning by analogy to the technique then being employed on a massive scale

against smallpox. This medico-historical literature attracted considerable attention in Britain. For the plague of 1770-72 reopened a basic question: was the disease contagious and, if it was, how might Britain protect herself against importing it via commerce with plague-endemic regions? Continuing British concern with this question helps account for the translation, however belatedly, of Mertens' book into English.

As a supplement to the republication of Mertens' account, this essay seeks to explore British responses to the plague, for they foreshadow the widespread European interest in the book. British diplomatic and press reports provide the documentary base of the study, though the reactions of other nations are also mentioned. Following brief discussions of the nature of bubonic plague, the Moscow epidemic and its comparison to the London plague of 1665, the bulk of the essay will examine British actions and commentaries in response to the medical menace of 1770-72 in Russia. A bibliography of works on plague in general and the Moscow epidemic in particular is appended to assist readers who wish to pursue these subjects further.

I.

For an occurrence that attracted widespread European interest for several decades, the epidemic that climaxed in Moscow in 1771 has been nearly forgotten. Several recent works even call it an outbreak of cholera or smallpox.[4] While other diseases may have been present, there can be no doubt that the main malady involved was bubonic plague. The origin of the epidemic southwest of Russian borders, its spread northward into the Ukraine and Russia, its development and apogee in Moscow, the clinical descriptions of contemporary medical and nonmedical observers--all concur with the established bionomics and etiology of bubonic plague.

As presently understood, bubonic plague is primarily a disease of wild
rodents caused by the bacterium <u>Pasteurella</u> <u>pestis</u> and transmitted by flea-
bite. Many species of rodents are susceptible to this pathogen, and thus
plague epizootics greatly outnumber epidemics; for the rodents bear more
fleas than people do and associate more intimately with their own kind than
with man. For an epidemic to occur, infected rodents bearing abundant
fleas must become numerous and live close to substantial aggregations of
people. Such a conjunction of circumstances rarely happens in conditions
of modern sanitation in the developed regions of the world. In previous
centuries, though, most urban inhabitants resided in multifamily wooden
houses that were infested with black rats (<u>Rattus</u> <u>rattus</u>). This species of
rodent prefers to live close to humans, from whose garbage and foodstuffs
it obtains nourishment and in whose dwellings it finds shelter. It breeds
rapidly and harbors fleas in great numbers, one species of which, <u>Xenopsylla</u>
<u>cheopis</u>, is an exceptionally efficient vector of plague. <u>R</u>. <u>rattus</u> is also
extraordinarily susceptible to infection by <u>P</u>. <u>pestis</u>; the blood of rats
dead from plague has been found to contain up to 100 million bacilli per
cubic millimeter. So when a black rat becomes infected with plague, some
of its fleas--<u>X</u>. <u>cheopis</u> above all--become infected too. The bacteria multiply and block the flea's feeding mechanism, causing the insect to become
ravenous. When its rodent-host dies of plague, the "blocked" flea seeks a
new host and, if human beings are within reach, attacks them. Unable to
ingest blood because its forestomach is blocked, the flea regurgitates
bacteria-laden matter into each skin puncture.

The bacteria injected into the human victim flow to the nearest lymph
glands, which become swollen as they battle the intruding germs. Such
swelling--the bubo--may occur wherever there are lymph glands, but it usually
appears on the neck, armpit or groin (the term bubo comes from the Greek

for groin). Occasionally the bacteria multiply so rapidly in the blood-
stream that they overwhelm the body's defenses before any swellings or
markings become visible; such a variation is termed septicemic plague. Less
often, the bacteria involve the lungs and cause primary pneumonic or pul-
monary plague. Pneumonic plague, unlike the bubonic form, can be transmitted directly from person to person without rat or flea intermediaries.
Pneumonic and septicemic plague kill virtually all their victims, unless
antibiotics are applied within hours of the disease's onset; whereas un-
treated bubonic plague usually kills 50-80 per cent of those infected within
a period of five days or more. Fortunately, pneumonic and septicemic plague
rarely occur and they tend to be self-limiting, as many victims perish before
they can pass on the malady. Bubonic plague, on the other hand, unfolds
more slowly and surreptitiously, beginning with an urban rat epizootic which
is then transmitted to humans by haphazard rat and flea contacts. The disease exhibits a marked seasonality, flourishing in warm and moderately moist
conditions. In temperate climates it ordinarily happens in the period from
spring to fall. As a rule cold weather cuts off an epidemic, for the fleas
hibernate and thereby break the chain of transmission. Neither the bionomics nor the etiology of plague was known before the first decade of the
twentieth century. The mysterious workings of the disease, its seemingly
arbitrary selection of victims, amplified the terror its visitations inspired. These facts about plague need to be kept in mind when considering
the pestilence of 1770-72 and the responses it evoked.[5]

Prior to 1770 Russia had suffered multiple visitations of plague, beginning with the Black Death of the mid-fourteenth century. Yet the epidemic
that erupted that year still surprised everybody. Epidemic plague had not
struck Russia for some thirty years and Russians, like the citizenry of

western Europe, had come to think of plague as a relic of the past. Few
medical practitioners in Russian service in 1770 had ever seen a case of
plague. In this regard Dr. Charles de Mertens (1737-1788) was no exception.
A native of Brussels, Mertens had studied medicine at Paris and Strasbourg
(M.D., 1758) and had practiced in Vienna before entering Russian service in
1767 (his name is also given as Karl or Carl von Mertens). He was hired
to attend the Foundling Home that Catherine II had established in Moscow
in 1763, and in 1768 he assisted in the introduction of the new Sutton-
Dimsdale method of inoculation against smallpox--a medical procedure that
Catherine personally underwent and vigorously publicized for her subjects.[6]
Evidently the empress had a hand in hiring Dr. Mertens.[7] At any rate she
probably met him while she was in Moscow for the legislative commission from
mid-1767 to early 1768, and she showed great confidence in his medical exper-
tise during his sojourn in Russia, which he left in 1772. Mertens resided
in Moscow throughout the pestilence of 1770-72. He participated in many
consultations of the city's physicians to discuss the disease and to recommend countermeasures. Though he had not seen plague before, he was well
qualified to write an account of it, having published a dissertation on the
epidemics of fever and dysentery that he observed at Vienna in 1762-63
(Vienna, 1766).[8] Thus Mertens brought to his analysis of the plague in
Moscow professional training in western Europe, practical experience in
Austria and Russia, and personal observation. These qualifications com-
pensated for his lack of previous direct experience with plague.

One reason the plague of 1770-72 surprised people in Russia was because
it first appeared abroad, in the Turkish vassal principalities of Moldavia
and Wallachia. Whether it arose from endemic foci in the Danubian Principalities, or was brought there from elsewhere, remains uncertain. Most

contemporaries assumed the disease was imported from Constantinople, an infamous incubator and distributor of pestilence. However that may be, the disease infected the Russian occupation forces in Wallachia and Moldavia in the spring of 1770, but because it displayed confusing symptoms and threatened to disrupt military operations against the Turks, the outbreak was kept secret from the general Russian population. Precautions were taken to protect the army, however, and cordons of troops were stationed along the border between Moldavia and Poland to prevent the infection going northward. These measures seemed to suffice; the Russian soldiery in the field largely escaped the scourge, which nevertheless penetrated into southern Poland as well as Transylvania in the summer of 1770. The ravages of the epidemic outside Russia are but dimly known. Poland suffered severely, even if contemporary estimates of 150,000 to 250,000 deaths from plague seem obviously inflated or must refer to the mortality from all causes. Eighteen villages in Transylvania were struck, with 1,204 deaths out of 1,624 cases reported.[9]

The pestilence first manifested itself in the Russia Empire at Kiev, just across the Polish border and the site of military magazines, sometime in August 1770. As before, it easily passed by the military cordon, whose personnel were checking for sick persons and suspect goods, not rats or fleas. The epidemic clearly followed the main military supply and trade routes northward from Moldavia, probably transported in grain shipments, empty gunny sacks, war booty such as clothes, soldiers' knapsacks, and so forth. Another likely mode of transmission was in bales of raw wool brought by Greek merchants from Turkish territory into the Ukraine and thence to Moscow, the chief textile manufacturing and marketing center of the empire. Once the epidemic reached Kiev, where it killed about 4,000 persons (just as Mertens reports), the imperial authorities deployed cordons along the borders

of the provinces adjoining the Ukraine, but still withheld any public announcement of the peril. Other Ukrainian towns suffered ravages--Nezhin,
with its sizable colony of Greek merchants, was badly hit--yet the pestilence
at Kiev began to abate in November 1770. The imperial authorities evidently
hoped that the advent of winter would halt the northward march of the plague.
Their hopes proved empty, probably due to an unusually long and mild
autumn.[10]

Moscow, as Mertens notes, was ideally suited to import and sustain
pestilence. The empire's co-capital, most populous city, greatest inland
emporium, leading textile producer, military supply depot, and a city whose
multiplying and motley population lived almost exclusively in wooden, multifamily houses, Moscow seemed planned for a plague. Indeed, the metropolis
was so sprawling and loosely administered that the authorities did not perceive the plague when it arrived. Evidently P. pestis was brought to Moscow
by November 1770, if not before.[11] The course of the Moscow epidemic need
not be recounted here in detail; Mertens himself provides a concise and
generally accurate description. His account of the pestilence judiciously
links its vagaries to climatic changes. He records the helplessness of the
city authorities, medical and administrative alike, to curtail the spread
of the infection. He mentions the depopulation of Moscow from the massive
flight of the well-to-do and how, accordingly, the disease afflicted mainly
the poor. He briefly relates the climax of the epidemic, the so-called
"Plague Riot" of September 15-17, 1771, that resulted in the death of Archbishop Amvrosii and ended with bloody skirmishes between a mob and troops
using cannon. Even the mortality statistics Mertens cites--80,000 dead in
Moscow and more than 100,000 including its district--approximate those from
official Russian sources.[12] Considering Mertens' brief experience in Moscow

prior to the epidemic and his sparse knowledge of Russian, his picture of
the epidemic is amazingly accurate.

The Moscow plague of 1771 resembled other urban outbreaks of previous
and subsequent periods. For instance, it exhibited several features in
common with the outbreak in London in 1665. The official mortality statistics,
though imprecise and almost certainly understated, sketch the progress and
scope of the two outbreaks. Both sets of data reveal the statistical curve
characteristic of plague in temperate climates.[13]

Month	Moscow	London
April	744	
May	851	
June	1,099	590
July	1,708	6,137
August	7,268	17,036
September	21,401	26,230
October	17,561	14,375
November	5,235	3,449
December	805	590
Total Deaths	56,672	68,407

Both outbreaks peaked in the period August-October, Moscow losing more than
46,000 victims then as compared to more than 57,000 in London. The Moscow
epidemic developed more gradually than the London outbreak, probably because
of a late spring in Russia in 1771 and the Russian city's more sprawling
layout. Yet the death toll in both cities manifested sudden, explosive up-
surges that suggest the plague arose from multiple riverine foci of rat-
plague in each case.[14] Though an inland city, Moscow stands at a junction
of several rivers, and its topography has been shaped by the windings of

the Moskva River, which shares the city's name. As a function of their
similar settlement patterns, both cities suffered more casualties in the
suburbs, where the plague began in both cases, than in their central dis-
tricts. Since London in 1665 had a population of about 460,000 as compared
to Moscow's 250,000 a century later, the proportional incidence of the
Russian epidemic evidently surpassed that of its English predecessor. To
be sure, in both cases massive flight, concealment of corpses, and widespread
undercounting hinder exact computation and comparison.[15] Still it seems
clear that both Moscow in 1771 and London in 1665 underwent plagues of com-
parable magnitude. The London epidemic, however, occasioned no eruption of
violence like the Plague Riot in Moscow. Why not?

Social tensions afflicted London during the plague just as they did
Moscow, the English authorities feared violence might erupt at any moment,
and some resistance to authority and some looting did occur. The municipal
and royal administrations were in disarray, too, much as their counterparts
were in Moscow a century later. The municipal economy of London was also
paralyzed by the pestilence, but hunger did not threaten the English capital
as much as it did the Russian city. The amount of medical assistance, professional and amateur alike, made available to the populace of London and
Moscow seems roughly equal, or perhaps somewhat greater in the Russian case.
Yet professional medical care was still a relatively new development in
eighteenth-century Russia, and a large proportion of the medical practitioners in Russian service were of foreign origin.[16] Both these facts may have
fed nativist and anti-elitist feelings among the populace of Moscow. When
provoked by the inept antiplague efforts of the authorities in Petersburg--
officialdom in Moscow foresaw the violence and pled for greater administrative
flexibility to avoid it--the Muscovites reacted with three days of rioting.

Several Soviet scholars have contended that this violence represented an "antifeudal revolt." The rioters, they argue, aimed to overthrow the established regime and organized the outbreak beforehand.[17] Such contentions ring hollow. They exaggerate the extent and significance of the violence, just as they neglect its immediate stimuli and spontaneous genesis.

One signal difference between London and Moscow, however, was that the former had suffered repeated outbreaks of pestilence in the relatively recent past and had developed an impromptu organization for such occasions. The regular local administration assumed responsibility for implementing antiplague policies. If one must doubt Bell's affirmation that "The Plague, with its daily repetition of dread and its visible horror, numbed all mob instinct among the people," he rightly suggests that "It was a great gain that the magistrates, aldermen and parish officers set over the people were those to whom they were accustomed." For, Bell admits, "A spirit of revolt was seething below the apparent calm."[18] In Moscow in 1771, on the contrary, there was little or no tradition of municipal responsibility, corporate autonomy or civic consciousness. There were few instances of communal self-help until the catastrophic progress of the plague, in conjunction with the temporary collapse of the city administration--the governor-general of Moscow, Field Marshal P. S. Saltykov, left the city on the eve of the Plague Riot--forced the populace to fend for itself.

The antiplague policies instituted in London in 1665 closely resembled those later adopted in Moscow. They exacerbated an already strained situation in each instance. But in London such policies were neither new nor surprising. They were frequently employed, and they were implemented through the regular administration. In Moscow, by contrast, the plague called forth a whole series of new arrangements. Officials and medics were assigned to each police district of the city; the governor-general and a specially appointed deputy, Senator and General P. D. Eropkin, coordinated antiplague policies formulated in consultation with the local medical office and communicated from St. Petersburg. There was no community involvement until, on the eve of the rioting, several groups secured permission to establish and administer their own quarantines. That lack of community cooperation and participation had worsened the situation in Moscow was tacitly recognized by the authorities when, several weeks after the rioting, they established the Commission for the Prevention and Treatment of the Pestilential Infectious Distemper, which included, besides administrators and medical men, prominent local representatives of the clergy and merchantry.[19] Had such an organization existed earlier in Moscow, it might have defused or limited the tension that exploded into the Plague Riot.

One Soviet commentator has asserted, perversely, that the real saviors of the situation in Moscow were neither the officials nor the medical men, but the rioters: their violence compelled the authorities to relax the rigid and ineffective regime of compulsory quarantines.[20] This view cannot be sustained, however; for it ignores both the Moscow authorities' attempts to avoid violence and the high level of mortality that persisted past mid-October 1771, i.e., for several weeks after the violence. The Plague Riot did not even prompt Catherine to send Count G. G. Orlov to Moscow as her personal emissary to quiet the situation. He left Petersburg on September 21 and only learned of the violence enroute. The most the violence accomplished was to persuade Catherine to endorse a modified quarantine policy, but while this policy may have forestalled renewed violence, it hardly affected the course of the epidemic. Cold weather, not rioters, curtailed the plague in Moscow, a point well put by Mertens.

II.

If Mertens' account rests upon the inside information of a privileged foreign resident of Moscow, what did British contemporaries inside and out-side Russia make of the pestilence? What did the foreign embassies learn? How did their governments react? What did the press report?

Obtaining reliable news from such remote regions and about such a sensi-tive subject was further complicated, of course, by the Russian policy of secrecy. The imperial Russian government did not publicly acknowledge the existence of the epidemic in Poland until January 3, 1771, when its procla-mation denied that the disease had even entered the empire.[21] Neither of the two official gazettes in St. Petersburg and Moscow printed anything about the plague until it reached its height. The Moskovskie vedomosti (Moscow News), for instance, never mentioned plague in Russia throughout 1771, though it reprinted numerous reports of its ravages in Poland and, especially, Turkey.[22] Such official reticence explains why the foreign press, relying on published and private reports from points adjoining the afflicted regions, often obtained earlier and fuller information about the epidemic than did the diplomatic chanceries in Russia. Thus the embassies in St. Petersburg had to rely on rumors and unconfirmed reports. The Austrian and British embassies took particular interest in the matter; the former because of its propinquity to the afflicted region and its designs on Polish territory, the latter because of its commercial interests in the Baltic and the Mediterranean.

On April 6, 1770, the Austrian embassy in Petersburg reported to Vienna that sickness among the troops of the Russian Second Army would delay the projected siege of Bender, a Turkish fortress on the lower Dniester. At the end of May the same source said that disease was hampering the spring cam-paigns of both Russian armies. A month later the Austrians learned that a

special medical observer (Dr. Johann Lerche) had been sent to investigate the
soaring mortality among the Russian soldiery in the south. Yet only on
August 17, 1770, did the Austrian diplomats in Petersburg confirm the existence of the epidemic in southern Poland and its spread toward Kiev. Austrian
authorities had meanwhile already activated the sanitary cordon along their
borders with the Ottoman Empire, and in late July they occupied several dis-
tricts of southern Poland in preparation for that country's partition. By
October 26 the Austrian representative in Petersburg knew that plague was
ravaging Kiev, and he remarked upon the strict official secrecy that shrouded
the subject. When the first Russian proclamation finally appeared on January 3, 1771, the Austrian embassy had already heard about some deaths in
the environs of Moscow.[23]

Like its Austrian counterpart, the British embassy in Petersburg secured
some vague reports of epidemics in the Russian armies occupying Moldavia and
Wallachia. "The Epidemical Distemper with which those Provinces have been
affected," reported Lord Cathcart, the British envoy, on July 16, 1770,
"and to which I have heard they are subject in the Spring is said to be
abated and not to affect the Troops in Camp, where every precaution is taken
to preserve the Health of the Soldiery: it would indeed be very unfortunate
if the same disorder were according to reports to extend itself to other
Territorys." Four days later the same observer relayed news about the operations of General Peter Panin's army against Bender: "there are those who
say that an Epidemical and Infectious Distemper rages in that Town and
neighborhood which has hitherto obliged the General to delay, but I cannot
assure Your Lordship of the Truth." Although Cathcart's forebodings about
the spread of the disease proved amply justified, he forwarded no more news
about it to London for the next eight months. Unlike the Austrian representative, he did not immediately report the initial outbreak in Moscow at the

end of 1770, only mentioning it on April 12, 1771, when he confirmed its recrudescence the previous month. He accepted Russian assurances that the disease had not been plague in either case.[24]

Despite Cathcart's reservations and reassurances, the British government received alarming reports from other quarters. The press seemed to know more about the epidemic than did the diplomatic chanceries, but it also published contradictory news. Citing a report from Warsaw of July 28, for example, the official London Gazette concluded on August 18 that "The best Accounts from Kaminiec and those Quarters assure us, that the Distemper which rages there is not the Plague, but a putrid Fever, which does not appear to be so general or destructive as was at first represented."[25] By contrast, the Scots Magazine at the same time carried reports of plague in Constantinople, Moldavia, Transylvania, and southern Poland. A report from Vienna on August 8, however, left "not the least doubt of the plague's raging in Moldavia."[26] Letters from Poland, relayed from Regensburg on August 17, "bring us very afflicting accounts. It is but too true, that the distemper of which so many have died in Podolia and Volhinia, and which was at first taken for a malignant fever, is really the plague; and that the contagion is spread into Transylvania, and even to Cronstadt."[27] Some suspected the epidemic might spread further. A report of August 4 from Vienna mentioned the plague in southern Poland and the reinforcement of the Austrian cordon against it. Yet the civil war in Poland, opined this observer, "will render all the precautions made use of upon such occasions abortive. The Russian armies will likewise find it very difficult to escape this distemper, on account of the indispensable communication which the carrying of provisions occasions."[28]

British public opinion appeared to anticipate the plague of 1770-72. London's experience with plague in 1665, the great fear and outpouring of journalism and medical theorizing that the Marseilles epidemic of 1720-22 had provoked in England, the popularity of Daniel Defoe's fictional _Journal of the Plague Year_ (1722)--all conditioned an early and intense response from British commentators to reports of the plague in southeastern Europe.[29] In February 1770 the editor of the _London Magazine_, explaining why he was printing an "Essay on Putrid Fevers, by Dr. Tissot," commented that "As few periods have been known in which putrid fevers were more fatal than the present, the following essay . . . must doubtless be highly agreeable to our readers."[30] The article did not distinguish plague from other sorts of fever, however.

Announcement in early October 1770 of a quarantine against shipping from the Baltic and the Mediterranean elicited additional comment. The _Universal Magazine_ inserted a poem "On War and Pestilence among the Turks." The _Weekly Magazine_ published a recipe "called the _Thieves Vinegar_, having been made use of by some abandoned wretches, who plundered the dying and the dead, in one of the great plagues abroad."[31] Several publications issued an item entitled "Hints Calculated to prevent the Plague spreading from other countries into this Kingdom," which advocated the construction of lazarets at the main ports for the reception and quarantine of suspect goods and persons. "We must be particularly careful to destroy the cloaths of the sick, because they harbour the very quintescence of contagion." Cotton was especially dangerous, the anonymous writer concluded, "and Turky is almost a perpetual seminary of the plague."[32]

Reports of the plague abroad inspired comparisons with the London outbreak of 1665, one account of which explained that "by seeing and correcting

the Errors and Mistakes of our Ancestors, we may, should we be visited
with the tremendous Scourge, in some Degree avoid or lessen the Horror and
Confusion in those Times." The same commentator closed his account with an
hysterical admonition:

> Can there be any thing more terrible? The very Stench of it
> will send thousands to their Graves, change Mansion-Houses into
> Pest-Houses, and gather Congregations into Church-Yards instead
> of Churches. Every Disease turns into the Plague; the very Breath
> infects. Of all the Miseries which can happen upon this Earth,
> this is the Horror! Art and Medicine are entirely useless;
> nothing can resist, nor stop the irresistable Stroke. No Age,
> Sex, or Condition is spared; the Cottage and the Palace alike are
> visited; the Rich and the Poor, the wise Man and the Fool, the
> Brave and the Coward, the Slave and his Lord, fall undistinguished;
> Men of Strength and in perfect Health are equally taken away with
> the aged and infirm; the People died not only with, but without
> the Infection, by Fear and Surprise. Melancholy and Despondency
> pry upon the Minds of many; Fearfulness and an horrible Dread seize
> upon all. Think on this, ye Ministers of State, and prevent,
> if possible, the Effects of so direful a Calamity! Let Repentance
> and Amendment of Life, o ye People, be your Charms to avert the
> poisoned Arrows of Death. [33]

Another analyst, having recounted the London outbreak, remarked that
"Plagues in this country are rather to be deemed accidental than original,
being generally brought from abroad by goods imported from infected places."
"Would it not be humane and generous in the college of physicians, at this
alarming crisis," the same writer wondered, apropos of the quackery and

nostrums popular a century before, "to prescribe and publish some cheap and salutary medicines for the benefit of the poor, to prevent or cure infection?"[34]

Even though the initial plague scare dissipated within a few months, comment continued into the new year, 1771, as the Weekly Magazine printed "A Strange Account of the Introduction of Plague into Poland," which maintained that the disease had arrived there in a letter from a merchant in the Levant to his wife. The woman allegedly kissed her husband's letter, fell ill that very night, and died in three days along with three others in her household. This story supported one popularly believed theory of infection: "It is very certain, that, while a person is writing a letter, their breath has such effect on the paper as to damp it, which being immediately folded up, must certainly retain the infection." "If I had any power," concluded "Meanwell," "not a letter should come into this Kingdom, without being pricked full of holes, and put in a sulphureous place for several days."[35] Lest this proposal seem idiosyncratic, it should be noted that the Russian government and many others also feared the spread of infection via postal communications, and endeavored to detour couriers around suspect regions and to fumigate dispatches.

Animated by stories of the plague, the royal government acted on some of the sentiments expressed in the press. On October 5, 1770, the British authorities declared a quarantine on shipping from the northeastern Baltic and also prohibited cattle imports from France because of an epizootic raging among the horned cattle on the continent.[36] British quarantine legislation, as codified in the statute of 1754, required shipments from the designated region to wait forty days from the time of arrival before unloading, to submit to medical inspection, and to air the goods for two weeks.

Concealment of plague on board carried the death penalty for the commander.[37]
Two weeks later the quarantine was broadened to include ships from the
Mediterranean as well as all shipments of rags and raw cotton, the latter
as "Goods more especially liable to retain Infection." Because of the continuing cattle plague, all hay and straw from the continent were ordered
to be burned. On November 1 the king in council extended the quarantine on
Baltic shipping to cargoes from Hamburg and Bremen. Swedish authorities also
announced in the British press on November 12 a quarantine requiring bills
of health from all persons and cargoes entering Sweden, in consequence of
"the Plague raging in the Levant and some Parts of Europe." Toward the end
of the month, however, British merchants trading with Hamburg and Bremen
petitioned for removal of the quarantine. The royal authorities granted their
request on November 30, except as it applied to shipments of rags and raw
cotton. Yet on December 9 the quarantine was reimposed because "His Majesty
hath received Information, that Hemp, and Flax, and Human Hair, and Feathers,
are frequently brought on board Ships coming from Hamburgh and Bremen,
which Goods are likewise more especially liable to retain Infection."[38]

The British quarantine on shipping from the Baltic lasted until May 24,
1771, when the king in council removed the restrictions in response to a
petition from merchants trading with the region and with assurances from
authorities in Königsberg, Riga, Narva, and Danzig that the plague had
ceased in the south. The restrictions on ships from Bremen and Hamburg were
lifted the same day for the same reason. Besides, the quarantine scarcely
affected British trade with the Baltic, for an unusually severe winter
shortened the shipping season and delayed its opening till the late spring.
The royal government also felt encouraged by an announcement of the Danish
authorities, on May 3, that reiterated their policy of inspecting ships from

the eastern Baltic, for fear that "the contagious Distemper, which appeared
in Poland and other places, (though diminished by the Severity of the Winter)
might resume its Force, and spread itself again, during the Spring and the
approaching Summer."[39]

Just as merchants in Britain urged the removal of their government's
quarantine, so the Russian authorities and the British mercantile community
in Russia sought to assuage fears of the plague's recrudescence. An anonymous report from Petersburg on December 28, 1770, denied that the plague had
hit the Russian army at Bender or had ever afflicted the Ukraine. "That
fatal Distemper never reached either of those Places. What gave Rise to the
Report was, that a Spotted Fever raged in several Places, which had the
Appearance of the Plague." The Russian ambassador in London likewise re-
assured the British public. Quoting recent letters from Russia, he publicly
announced on February 23, 1771, "there is not (thank God) the least appearance of any infectious Distemper, either in Moscow, Livonia, Estonia, Ingria,
or in the adjacent Provinces; and . . . the Measures taken to prevent its
being introduced into them, leave not the least Reason to apprehend, in
future, any Danger from it." Nor did the foreign press immediately question
such reports. The same issue that carried the Russian ambassador's assurances relayed without comment an advice from The Hague, dated February 15:
"The Report which prevailed here of the Plague's having broken out at Moscow,
is formally contradicted by the Letters received this Morning from Petersburg." Toward the end of May news from Hamburg endorsed this conclusion.[40]

Equally soothing to British apprehensions about plague in Russia was
an extract of a letter from Petersburg, dated April 12, that obviously
emanated from British mercantile circles. "You may rest assured," the anonymous correspondent averred, "every thing is as well here as can be wished;

and should you hear any vague report about Moscow, desire you will pay as little attention to it as we do here, the alarm being without foundation, and every thing equally well there." Quarantine precautions were unnecessary in the port of Petersburg, the same report continued, because the goods for export were being inspected enroute from the interior, "more by way of prevention than any known or real cause; and I hope will have its proper weight with you, and other parts abroad."[41] These reassurances received authoritative support from Lord Cathcart. The plague could not be in Moscow, he was confident, for "fewer People have died there this Spring than has ever been remembred." Nevertheless, the quarantine between Moscow and Petersburg was being continued "to prevent any alarm being suddenly taken here which might create great Detriment to Commerce by being propogated and occasioning Quarantines on foreign Ports upon Vessels freighted from hence."[42]

Till late August 1771 British representatives in Russia reported nothing more about the plague. If they secured information in the interim, they withheld it in hopes that, as before, the rumors of plague would prove false. Fears for the export trade prompted both the Russian government and the British community in Russia to exercise great caution in reporting anything about plague. Furthermore, the peculiar course of the epidemic at Moscow, the two apparently false alarms in late 1770 and early 1771, baffled contemporary observers and caused them to doubt the reality of the disease. As late as August 25, 1771, Catherine herself told her council that she still hoped it was not really plague. And when Count Orlov arrived in Moscow on September 26, the first question he asked was whether it was really plague.[43] Such doubts were not peculiar to the outbreak in Moscow; they arose elsewhere before and later. As L. F. Hirst remarks, "No name in medicine sounds so ominous as plague; none is so charged with mass emotion."[44]

Notwithstanding the official and private reticence about the epidemic
in Russia, the foreign press pertinaciously propagated reports of its re-
appearance there. From Danzig on June 25 came the news that pestilence had
broken out anew in Moldavia in May but had been stopped by quick countermeasures. On August 5 another report from Danzig confirmed the plague's
recrudescence: "it makes great ravages in the Ukraine, in Podolia, in the
palatinate of Russia, and has reached to within eight miles of Leopol."
Plague had reappeared in Turkey, too, causing hundreds of deaths daily at
Smyrna and infecting foreign vessels in the harbor. Rumor ran amuck, of
course, and evoked Russian denials as late as the last week of August.
"The Reports of the Plague, or a Distemper resembling it, being at Moscow,"
an advice from Petersburg insisted on August 27, "are without Foundation.
It is true there is a Fever there, which the poor Patients conceal till the
last Extremity, for Fear of being sent by the Police to the Pest-Houses,
which makes them appear to die suddenly. The Government have nevertheless
taken Precautions against its spreading." Lord Cathcart transmitted the
same news a day earlier, commenting: "As to the Plague at Moscow your Lordship may depend upon it, it has never existed: tho' many principal Inhabitants have deserted the Town, and the Government have from complicated reasons
of Policy, established a Quarantine."[45]

By early September, however, such optimism began to wilt. A letter
from Petersburg of September 13 admitted that "We are still in the most
cruel uncertainty as to the nature of the malady which reigns at Moscow,"
but added, hopefully: "A month's quarantine is already ordered, and other
precautions taken."[46] Once the Russian authorities concluded that the
epidemic at Moscow was really pestilential and admitted the fact--Lord
Cathcart reluctantly reached the same conclusion on September 20, 1771--near

panic gripped Petersburg. To calm the populace and to mollify the apprehensions of the mercantile community at home and abroad, the imperial government had the Petersburg police issue a proclamation on October 10 in Russian,
French, German, and Finnish that enacted an array of precautions; and on
October 14 the Senate announced a general augmentation of the quarantines
surrounding Petersburg. These measures, coupled with reports of the rapid
abatement of the epidemic in the last weeks of October, eased fears in
Petersburg by early November. Although the plague spread outward from Moscow, it never really threatened Petersburg.[47] "Vinegar is burnt in great
quantities in every house," William Richardson, the tutor of Lord Cathcart's
children, wrote from Petersburg on December 3, 1771; "and the utmost attention is paid to the health of the lower ranks. Yet it is not very pleasant
to be within two or three days journey of so dreadful a neighbour."[48] In
December 1771 Prince Lobkowitz, the Austrian ambassador, reported an outbreak at Novaia Ladoga, about 100 miles from Petersburg, but it must have
been either a false alarm or have dissipated shortly.[49] Cold weather saved
Petersburg.

The British response to this new crisis followed two different courses,
as it had before. British officials in Russia, led by ambassador Cathcart
and consul-general Samuel Swallow, who was also a member of the British
Factory or mercantile community of Petersburg, saw no reason to alter policy.
They continued to accept Russian assurances that there was no immediate
danger to commerce at Petersburg and therefore opposed any quarantine of
goods shipped from Russian ports. Russian officialdom was taking every precaution to safeguard merchandise brought to Petersburg for export, Cathcart
concluded on September 23; hence Swallow was still granting bills of health
to departing British ships, "this City as well as Cronstadt being entirely
free from any Contagious or Pestilential Distemper." Both Cathcart and

Swallow feared the epidemic would cause commercial paralysis in Moscow,
however, and thereby force Russian merchants to default on their obligations
to British and other foreign interests.[50] Cathcart eagerly dispatched news
of the lessening of the plague. He obviously hoped to forestall a British
quarantine of Russian goods, "certainly as yet unnecessary," he remarked on
November 18, unaware that the measure had been adopted three weeks earlier.
When, four days later, Cathcart learned of the quarantine order, he reiterated his belief: "I do not apprehend there has ever been the least Hazard
of the Plague's being brought to any of the Russian Sea Ports this Season."
Enclosed in this dispatch was a letter from the British Factory, signed by
representatives of fifteen firms, that also argued against a quarantine of
goods already shipped from Russia. Repeating the arguments that Cathcart had
marshalled, the merchants assured that "no danger is to be apprehended from
any Cargoes ship'd from hence this Season, the Navigation of which is now
entirely closed by the setting in of the Winter."[51] As in 1770, so in 1771
the British quarantine came too late to have any immediate effect on exports from Russia.

Authorities in London viewed the situation in a gloomier light than
did the British colony in Petersburg. Cathcart's dispatch of September 20
acknowledging the disease as plague and Swallow's of September 23 detail-
ing Russian quarantine practices reached London at the beginning of November, just as newspaper reports of the tragedy in Moscow had reached a cre-
scendo.[52] The Dutch envoy in Petersburg, it was reported on October 23,
had sent word that "the Plague has broke out at Moscow, and makes great
Havock there"; and authorities in Holland were said to be contemplating
"the necessary Steps to prevent the Communication of the Plague to the Terri-
tories of this Republick." Though a spokesman of the Russia Company publicly

denied these reports on October 25, a dispatch from Petersburg the very
next day contradicted his assurances that the disease was not plague but
"spotted fever." "The Accounts we receive from Moscow are very melancholy,"
reported the unnamed correspondent in Petersburg. "Great Numbers die daily
of a malignant Fever which prevails there, and which, as it appears to be
epidemical, the greatest Precautions are taking to prevent its spreading
further." A week later, on November 2, another advice from Petersburg
finally acknowledged the disease was plague.[53]

These diplomatic and press reports caused King George III to refer
the matter to the Privy Council, which on November 4 consulted with the
governor and several members of the Russia Company. The latter apparently
persuaded the councilors to delay the imposition of a quarantine until more
information could be obtained. So the council ordered Lord Suffolk, Secre-
tary of State for the Northern Department, to write Cathcart and Swallow at
once for complete accounts of the situation in Russia. Swallow might still
issue bills of health, the council directed, so long as he certified that
Petersburg was free of infection and that the goods in question had been
opened and aired before embarkation. Four days later, however, the king
joined the council to order a quarantine on all ships from Russian ports.[54]
Why the sudden reversal of the wait-and-see policy so recently adopted?

Alarming accounts appeared in the British press right after the council
meeting of November 4. The London Gazette on November 5 briefly described
the rioting in Moscow and reported that the Swedish government had established
a cordon in Finland. That same day an unsigned letter from Petersburg of
October 8 conveyed the following graphic details:

> The malignant Distemper which has broke out at Moscow,
> has caused great Disturbance and Confusion among the Common

People, which is the particular Reason why the Remedies and
Industry of the Physicians to stop its Progress have been
ineffectual; and by the following Account received from thence,
the 4th instant, the Populace have carried their Excesses to
the highest Pitch. Ambrosius, Archbishop of Moscow, perceiving
that many Abuses had crept in among the Common People, through
the Artifice of some designing Persons among them, thought it
his Duty to put a Stop to their Progress. These Imposters
found Means to collect the major Part of the People to one
of the City Gates, where there is an Image of the Virgin
Mary, and worked on their Credulity, by a false Appearance of
Religion, to gratify their own lucrative Intentions. The People,
even many of the Sick, came in vast Crouds to this Place, and
threw Money into a Chest put there for that Purpose, by which
Means the Distemper was spread surprisingly, and the Croud was
so great, that many People were trod to Death. To put a Stop
to such villainous and impious Practices, the Archbishop sent
proper Officers to seal up the Chest; but the blinded Multitude,
who looked upon this Action as a Disrespect to, and Disturbance
of their Religion, immediately gathered themselves together,
and plundered the Archbishop's House; but not finding him there,
they went to the Convent, where this worthy Archbishop was killed
by them in the most cruel and barbarous Manner. As soon as the
Government of Moscow heard that the People were in an Uproar,
they sent the Troops against them; by whose Hands many of
these Wretches fell victims to their own Credulity, and blind
Bigotry. A vast Number of them were taken Prisoners, who will
be punished as the Law directs for so great a Trespass.[55]

On November 7 another lengthy account of the Plague Riot appeared in the
same newspaper. This flurry of tremulous reports impelled the king in
council to proclaim, on November 8, 1771, a quarantine on all ships arriving from Russian ports.[56]

The British quarantine marked a renewal of the policy that had been in
force from October 5, 1770, to May 24, 1771. Like the earlier quarantine,
moreover, this one evoked efforts to repeal or modify it. Though the
British colony in Petersburg opposed the quarantine from the start, denounc-
ing it as both unnecessary and impossible to implement, it remained in effect
until September 10, 1772. Several circumstances prolonged this second
quarantine. For one, the king supported it. In a speech to Parliament on
January 21, 1772, George III discussed trade and foreign policy, remarking:
"The Danger of the farther Spreading of the infectious Sickness in Europe
is, I trust, very much abated. But I must recommend it to you not to suffer
our Happiness, in having been hitherto preserved from so dreadful a Calamity,
to lessen your Vigilance in the Use of every reasonable Precaution for our
Safety."[57] For another, the royal government felt constrained to follow
the lead of other maritime nations. Since the press carried reports of
Denmark, Sweden, and the Dutch Republic having adopted precautions, Britain
had to follow suit or risk retaliatory restrictions on her own shipping.[58]
And finally, the failure of British representatives abroad to provide timely
warning of the threat made their superiors in London doubly cautious.

Lord Suffolk explained the government's thinking to ambassador Cathcart
on January 31, 1772. The quarantine, he admitted, was irksome,

> But any Danger of the Plague must over ballance all other
> Considerations; and till the Distemper is totally eradicated,
> there can be no other Assurance of Safety. So long as a

Quarantine is continued in other Maritime Countries, it must
be maintained here, lest our Intercourse with those Countries
should be affected by the Neglect which would be imputed to Us:
And the Pains taken to propagate a Persuasion, that the Plague
was not at Moscow, when it was raging there, will, perhaps,
from the Doubts which will be entertained of all subsequent
Accounts, prolong the Quarantines; but their Rigour, & Duration,
will be abated, in Proportion as those Accounts may be
authenticated & favourable.[59]

Acting on the council order of November 4 to obtain trustworthy information about the plague and the Russian precautions against it, Cathcart and
Swallow plumbed various sources. They talked with Russian officials, obtained translations of the quarantine regulations, corresponded with informants
in Moscow, consulted members of the British Factory, investigated the origin
of Russian exports to Britain, read medical and historical treatises about
plague. While Russian officials proved eager to answer British inquiries,
the reluctant response of private sources made consul Swallow despair, "not
only from the difficulty of procuring true and circumstantial intelligence
from People in Trade here, but also from the restraint of those inhabiting
that City [Moscow], who are fearfull of touching upon the Subject in their
Letters."[60] Swallow's complaint had foundation. At the height of the pestilence Catherine restricted mail deliveries from Moscow and even burned some
French letters that termed the violence a "riot."[61] Still, by November 29,
1771, Swallow succeeded in compiling quite a full and accurate account of
the epidemic from its origins, a copy of which is appended to this essay.
This report reached London on January 3, 1772, and together with a letter
in French from Moscow that Swallow sent three weeks later, it provided all

the background information that the British government had requested. At
the turn of the year Cathcart also dispatched a disquisition on the plague
and its possible threat to British shipping.[62]

Cathcart and Swallow used all this "research" to defend their view that
a general quarantine of goods from Russia was not needed. They conceded,
however, that certain goods such as linen cloth might merit special attention.
Though they had failed to block the adoption of a general quarantine, its
declaration in November 1771 had little practical effect because the shipping
season had already ended. In concert with the British Factory, Cathcart
and Swallow pressed for a lifting of the quarantine when navigation reopened
in the spring of 1772 or, failing that, for the exclusion of certain goods--
hemp and flax in particular--from all or part of the quarantine period.
Swallow also informed Lord Suffolk that he could not implement the council
order to specify, on the bills of health he issued, the origin of the goods
being shipped. Merchandise came to Petersburg from all directions and from
great distances, he noted, and was often mixed together enroute.[63]

These arguments, and reports of the disappearance of the plague from
Moscow and elsewhere, did not change policy in London at once. Lord Suffolk
welcomed news of the end of the pestilence, but relayed rumors of epidemics in
the Crimea and predicted: "It will probably shew itself to the Southward
as the Summer advances, and wherever it appears in Russia it is an object
of attention." Cathcart's dispatch of April 6, 1772, announcing the plague
was over in the Crimea, was published in the London Gazette; but the government's lingering uncertainty shone forth anew at a meeting of the Privy
Council, on May 13, which approved the publication of a recipe for fumigatory
powders that the plague commission in Moscow had devised and which Cathcart
had forwarded on March 16. Lord Suffolk wrote Swallow on June 5 not to

expect any alteration of the quarantine till the warm season had passed.
Swallow replied on July 10 that there was no trace of plague in Russia,
particularly among consignments arriving at Petersburg from the interior,
and that he was granting bills of health as before. Yet the king in council
had already reaffirmed the quarantine on July 8, apprehending that warm
weather might regenerate the pestilence. At the end of August, moreover,
Lord Suffolk sent Swallow reports of plague in Poland. But this was the
last alarm.[64]

Swallow's dispatch of July 31 from Petersburg, which reached London
in early September, dispersed all remaining doubts. "There is not the least
symptom of the Plague from Jassy in Moldavia to this Place, to be found,"
wrote the British consul; "every Town & City within the boundaries of this
Empire, being in equal good Health with that which we have the Happiness
to enjoy here, as well as at the different Ports in the Baltick." And he
requested the Privy Council "to grant such ease & relief to the Trade from
this Country, as to them may seem meet." Accordingly, when the Russia
Company in London petitioned the government to abolish the quarantine, the
king in council approved the action on September 10, 1772. Raw cotton remained the only article still subject to quarantine.[65] The British quarantine of 1771-72, though it lasted nearly a year, had negligible effect on
the volume of Russian exports to Britain. Stung by experience, British representatives in Russia continued to watch for plague in subsequent years.
No further outbreaks threatened northern Europe directly, but periodic alarms
emanated from the Mediterranean, one of which prompted Dr. Richard Pearson
to translate Mertens' book in 1799.

III.

By way of a postscript, it may be mentioned that at least three British medical men witnessed the plague of 1770-72 firsthand. Their experiences add a further dimension to British responses to the epidemic. Indeed, one of them, George Smyth, allegedly survived "two different attacks of the plague, with all its characteristic symptoms, such as bubos, carbuncles, & c.," while serving as a surgeon with the Russian army.[66] Dr. Matthew Halliday (1732-1809) accompanied Count Orlov to Moscow in September 1771 and assisted in the last stages of the epidemic in that city. He was later sent to contain an outbreak at Yaroslavl. Few particulars of Halliday's service are known, except that he is supposed to have successfully used James's powder, an antimonial concoction popular at the time, against the disease.[67] Dr. Matthew Guthrie (1743-1807) may not have seen plague while at Russian headquarters in Jassy in 1772, at least he made no such claim. All the same, he took a scholarly interest in the subject, interviewed many army medical men who had treated the disease, and published a brief account of, and commentary upon, their findings. At the very end of his life he also penned a few unpublished reflections about the Moscow epidemic and Count Orlov's policies against the plague.

In his discussion of plague Guthrie, like Mertens before him, manifested the medical eclecticism of the age. Reflecting the then dominant contagionist theory, he contended that plague "may be rendered much less destructive than formerly, by a proper police, as it only is communicated by actual contact, or the touch, a fact firmly settled and determined when the pest was in Moscow." Plague did not spread through the air, as the miasmatic theory held; in Moscow it struck only "the infected multitude, who inoculated one another by the touch; no caution or persuasion having any effect on predestinarians either in Russia or Turkey." The wealthier social groups escaped entirely, "though they inhabited the upper storeys of the houses (to be more insulated and separated from the mob) and it is well known that corrupted, or mephitic air, being much lighter than common air mounts up; so of course if the plague had been communicated by the atmosphere, the inhabitants of the upper storeys could not have escaped as they did."[68] In contrast to Mertens' English translator, Dr. Pearson, who believed that various epidemic diseases could become pestilential, Guthrie distinguished plague "from the worst sort of malignant fever in hot countries." He also argued against the traditional forty-day quarantine in favor of a three-week period, "made more effectual by bathing and well cleaning the body with soap and water, so as to remove every adhering particle." A shorter quarantine might actually strengthen the effectiveness of the whole procedure, he thought, by lessening the temptation to violate the period of isolation.[69]

The Moscow plague, and Mertens' account of it, contributed to the ongoing European debate about the nature of the dread disease. Mertens interpreted plague from a cautiously miasmatico-contagionist perspective, emphasizing contact as the main mode of transmission. Nevertheless, he conceded that the air around a plague victim might become infected and counseled attending physicians to guard against air-borne transmission. Like all the other medical writers who published accounts of the Moscow epidemic, he did not link plague to any sort of rodent or micro-organism. Mertens' treatise became known in British medical circles well before his book was translated. Thus Dr. John Haygarth recommended the French edition of 1784 to John Howard, in June 1789, when the latter was embarking on his second (and last) trip to Russia. "This treatise of Dr. <u>Mertens</u> is in many respects excellent," concluded Haygarth.[70] Recent research also affirms the justice of this judgment.[71]

John T. Alexander

University of Kansas

1977

Appendix

Samuel Swallow's Report of the Plague in Russia
St. Petersburg, November 29/December 10, 1771

I had this day See'night the honour of writing your Lordship, with
translation of an Edict published by the Senate, regulating the several
Quarantines to be observ'd in forwarding Goods to the different Ports of
this Empire, & proceed now to communicate such further intelligence as
have hitherto been able to collect --

In the first Campaign An. 1769. after the Army got a footing in
Moldavia by taking Choczim, & the subsequent reduction of other Places,
the Plague discover'd itself in several of the Russian Detachments, & in
the Spring following An. 1770. rag'd with great violence at Iassi, the then
head Quarters of Field Marchall Count Rumantzoff, but almost totally dis-
appear'd upon the Army taking the Field. As however the Disorder existed
more or less in almost every corner of those newly conquer'd Provinces, &
the communication so frequent with the southern parts of Poland & the
Ukrain, it soon found its way, first into the one & then into the other,
& in Autumn & the succeeding Winter 1770. rag'd with destructive Violence
at Kioff & the adjacent Country.

In or about December last there was an alarm that the Plague had
appear'd at Mosco, from the sudden Death of some Workmen in a Cloth Fabrick,
but was never properly determin'd whether it was the real Pestilential Disorder or not, & as it entirely subsided for some Months, People got entirely
the better of their Fears, and believ'd it to be a ridiculous Chimera. In
the month of June however it began again to appear amongst the Cloth workers,
and during July & August, before it was properly attended to, spread its
banefull influence so wide, that many different Quarters of that extensive

City were affected, & many numerous Family's of the lower class, were almost totally rooted out.

Altho' different causes are assigned; yet according to the best information I have been able to procure, the infection was brought to Mosco from Brahiloff in Moldavia the begining of last Winter, in a quantity of Wool which was sold to the Cloth Fabrick aforemention'd, and it is also imputed to the Servants of General Stoffels, having after their Masters Death, brought some of his Apparel to Moscow (supposed to have been infected) & sold it at the publick Market.

The Distemper was at its heighth in the latter end of September & begining of October, when from seven to Nine Hundred People Died in a day, & has also spread in the adjacent Country, partly by their frequent communication with the City, partly by the Flight of many People concern'd in the late Tumult, & partly by several of those employ'd in the Fabricks, taking advantage of the short Anarchy that then prevail'd, to return to the Villages to which they belong'd, which is presum'd to be the cause of its having extended to Jeroslaw, & several of the neighbouring Villages, as well as Kaluga, where it is however said to be entirely suppress'd, & the same good intelligence is shortly expected from Jeroslaw, by the wise Conduct of the principal Inhabitants, upon its first appearance there. --

The City of Mosco from its opulence & situation, is the Mart for furnishing the other inland Towns & Citys of the Empire with all sorts of Foreign Goods imported at this & other Ports on the Baltick, as well as Silks & other Commodity's which before the Warr, were sent thither from Dantzig & Königsberg through Poland, but an entire stop has been put thereto since last Winter, and 'till Health is again restor'd, no Goods or Merchandize whatsoever are allowed to be sent out of that unhappy City, neither is

anything permitted to be brought in, but what is necessary for the support
of the Inhabitants, so that several sorts of Russia Products brought hither
by Land, which formerly us'd to pass through Mosco, are now oblig'd to come
by different Roads, some at the distance of 20. & others at 50. to 100.
Versts, according to the situation of the respective Citys from whence the
Goods are originally sent & which in effect is consider'd as a Cordon to
prevent the infection from spreading elsewhere, there being Quarantines
establish'd at all the Places within those distances round Moscow, to pro-
hibit any Person or Goods from going nearer, unless intended for the use
of the City, & further no Person is allow'd to travel from one Place to the
other, without Bills of Health, or performing a regular Quarantine, as will
be more clearly seen by referring to the Edict lately publish'd by the
Senate on that head, by which it also appears (the same regulations having
been in part observed last Winter) that even during the course of this, as
well as next Year, the requisite precautions for examining & purifying the
Goods were, & will be taken & observed before they reach this Place,
Archangel, Reval or Riga; & a better proof cannot well be given of the Goods
already exported having undergone such an examination as well as of their
purity, before & after they arrived at this Port, than that not a single
Person accompanying or employ'd in the opening, assorting, or repacking
them, at the time they were to be ship'd, has been in any shape affected
thereby or receiv'd any Disorder whatsoever, tho' many in number, & their
daily employment during the Shiping Season. These were the reasons which
induc'd me to continue granting Bills of Health to all Ships going from hence,
being fully persuaded (as I then was) that their Cargoes were entirely free
from infection.

Count Orloff return'd last Friday Evening to his House at Gatchina about 50. Versts from hence, where His Excellency is to perform thirty Days Quarantine, & during his residence at Moscow establish'd two Commissions. The first, composed of General Yeropkin a Senator, three Physicians, two Surgeons & other Assistants, to inspect & order such regulations as would be found most eligible to relieve and provide for all Persons who were infected with the Distemper, to prevent any one from having communication with them, but such as were appointed by the Commission, & that proper care should be taken in burying the Dead, and burning their Apparel & c.

The second Commission, wherein the Senator Wolkoff & Master of the Police preside, are to see that all such Orders and Regulations as the first may judge necessary, be duly & properly executed, both to the relief of the sick & to prevent the infection from being communicated to others, that they shall both decide immediately upon all Cases brought before them, without going through the forms of other Courts of Justice, and daily notify to each other every occurrence that happens; beside which they are also jointly to report a circumstantial Account of all to the Senate in Mosco, & there is reason to believe the operations of these Commissions, together with the Frost continuing, have greatly contributed to the decrease of the Disease, as it manifestly has, to the maintaining good Order and Tranquility within the City. In a Letter from thence received by the last Mail, a Correspondent of mine uses the following words "we begin to entertain good Hopes that the Epidemium will be totally eradicated in the course of the Winter as it abates very much," and it is further said here, the number of Deaths in a Day are diminished to about Sixty, but as no regular Lists are publish'd, cannot take upon me to assure Your Lordship of these reports being exact.

I hope soon to procure a translation of the Instructions to Count Bruce, who has the general Command over all the Quarantines, in the mean time

have the honour to convey to Your Lordship a Publication of the Police of
this City, instructing the Inhabitants how to behave on the present Occasion;
& also a translation of an Ukaze from the Senate by which all Merchants
except His Majesty's Subjects (who are to pay as stipulated by the Treaty
of Commerce) & Russians, are henceforth to pay their Duty's in Rix Dollars
the same as before the Tariff at present existing, was form'd.

I just now learn the epidemical Distemper had made its Appearance at
Tula, but by enclosing the few Houses infected, which with the Cloaths &
other materials were afterwards burnt, & removing the People to proper
Lazarets, (the method at present adopted,) it was as suddenly suppress'd,
& the Town is again in Health, which is of great consequence, as beside many
wealthy Merchants who live there, the chiefest part of the Inhabitants are
employ'd in making arms for the Government.

Your Lordship may depend on my transmiting whatever else may come to
my Knowledge on this calamitous & interesting Subject, . . .

Source: PROSP, 91/88, pp. 291-94v.

Notes

The research for this article was supported in part by NIH Grant
1 R01 LM 01664-01, from the National Library of Medicine, and by grants
from the General Research Fund, the Graduate School, and the Faculty Development Fund of the University of Kansas. For critical reviews of an earlier
draft, I am grateful to my colleagues Clifford Griffin, Norman Saul, and
Richard Sheridan. Materials emanating from Russia are dated by the Julian
Calendar, which in the eighteenth century lagged eleven days behind the
Gregorian Calendar used in the rest of Europe.

1. Albert Sorel, The Eastern Question in the Eighteenth Century, trans.
F. C. Bramwell (London, 1898; reprinted New York, 1969); Herbert H. Kaplan,
The First Partition of Poland (New York and London, 1962).

2. Erik Amburger, Russland und Schweden 1762-1772 (Berlin, 1934; reprinted
Vaduz, 1965); Robert R. Palmer, The Age of the Democratic Revolution: A
Political History of Europe and America, 1760-1800, vol. 1, The Challenge
(Princeton, 1959), pp. 85-103, 164-173.

3. Sorel, pp. 108-109; Kaplan, pp. 129-130; Amburger, pp. 245-246.

4. Miriam Kochan, Life in Russia under Catherine the Great (London and
New York, 1969), p. 138; Paul Avrich, Russian Rebels, 1600-1800 (New York,
1972), p. 222; Robert Coughlan, Elizabeth and Catherine (New York, 1974),
p. 269.

5. J. F. B. Shrewsbury, A History of Bubonic Plague in the British Isles
(Cambridge, 1970), pp. 1-17; K. F. Meyer, "Pasteurella and Francisella,"
in Rene J. Dubois and James G. Hirsch, eds., Bacterial and Mycotic Infections
of Man, 4th ed. (Philadelphia and Montreal, 1965), pp. 664-677.

6. Philip H. Clendenning, "Dr. Thomas Dimsdale and Smallpox Inoculation in
Russia," Journal of the History of Medicine and Allied Sciences, vol. 27,
no. 2 (April 1973), 109-125, and W. J. Bishop, "Thomas Dimsdale, M.D., F.R.S.

(1712-1800) and the Inoculation of Catherine the Great of Russia," Annals of Medical History, n.s., vol. 4, no. 4 (July 1932), 321-338.

7. Ia. A. Chistovich, Istoriia pervykh meditsinskikh shkol v Rossii (St. Petersburg, 1883), app. X, pp. ccxv-ccxvi.

8. Biographisches Lexikon der hervorragenden Ärzte aller Zeiten und Völker, 2nd ed. (Berlin and Vienna, 1932), vol. 4, p. 178.

9. Georg Sticker, Abhandlungen aus der Seuchengeschichte und Seuchenlehre, vol. 1: Die Pest, pt. 1 (Giessen, 1908), pp. 252-259; Moskovskie vedomosti (Moscow), May 3, 1771, citing a report from "the Lower Elbe," April 1, 1771.

10. A. Andreevskii, "Arkhivnaia spravka o morovoi iazve v g. Kieve v 1770-1771 gg.," Kievskaia starina, vol. 34 (July 1891), 304-314.

11. [A. F. Shafonskii], Opisanie morovoi iazvy, byvshei v stolichnom gorode Moskve s 1770, po 1772 god, s prilozhenie vsekh dlia prekrashcheniia onoi togda ustanovlennykh uchrezhdenii (St. Petersburg, 1787), pp. vi-vii, 40-41.

12. Ibid., 601.

13. Ibid., 601; Shrewsbury, p. 462.

14. Shrewsbury, p. 462.

15. W. G. Bell, The Great Plague in London in 1665 (London and New York, 1924), pp. 12, 20.

16. A. Brückner, Die Aerzte in Russland bis zum Jahre 1800 (St. Petersburg, 1887). See also Heinz Müller-Dietz, Der russische Militärarzt im 18. Jahrhundert (Berlin, 1970) and idem., Ärzte im Russland des achtzehnten Jahrhunderts (Esslingen/Neckar, 1973).

17. P. K. Alefirenko, "Chumnyi bunt v Moskve v 1771 godu," Voprosy istorii, no. 4 (April 1947), 82-88; V. N. Bernadskii, "Ocherki iz istorii klassovoi bor'by i obshchestvenno-politicheskoi mysli Rossii v tret'ei chetverti XVIII veka," Uchenye zapiski Leningradskii gos. ped. inst. im. A. I. Gertsena, vol. 229 (1962), pp. 94-98.

18. Bell, pp. 173-175.

19. Shafonskii, pp. 55-58, 100-101 et passim.

20. Alefirenko, p. 87.

21. Polnoe sobranie zakonov rossiiskoi imperii, 1st.Ser. (St. Petersburg, 1830), vol. 19, no. 13, 551.

22. See, for example, Moskovskie vedomosti, 1 April, 3 May, 6 May, 30 Aug. 1771, etc.

23. Seddler to Kaunitz, 6 April, 25 May, 22 June, 29 June, 17 August, 26 October 1770, 4 Jan. 1771, Sbornik imperatorskogo russkogo istoricheskogo obshchestva, 148 vols. (1870-1916), vol. 109 (St. Petersburg, 1901), pp. 437, 445, 450-51, 460-61, 478 -- hereafter cited as SIRIO; Sorel, p. 97. See also Gunther E. Rothenberg, "The Austrian Sanitary Cordon and the Control of Bubonic Plague: 1710-1871," Journal of the History of Medicine and Allied Sciences, vol. 28, no. 1 (Jan. 1973), 15-23.

24. Cathcart to Wroughton, 16 July 1770; Cathcart to Rochford, 20 July 1770, Public Record Office, State Papers, 91/85, pp. 57v., 79v.-80--hereafter cited as PROSP; Cathcart to Halifax, 1 April 1771, SIRIO, vol. 19, p. 205; Cathcart to Halifax, 19 April 1771, PROSP, 91/87, p. 190v.

25. London Gazette, Aug. 18, 1770.

26. Scots Magazine (Edinburgh), Aug. 1770, pp. 444, 447.

27. Ibid., Sept. 1770, p. 506.

28. The London Magazine, or Gentleman's Monthly Intelligencer, Sept. 1770, p. 491.

29. Charles F. Mullett, The Bubonic Plague and England (Lexington, Kentucky, 1956), pp. 251-334.

30. London Magazine, Feb. 1770, pp. 93-96.

31. The Universal Magazine of Knowledge and Pleasure (London), Oct. 1770,
pp. 214-215, 217-218; The Weekly Magazine or Edinburgh Amusement, Oct. 18,
1770, p. 115.

32. Weekly Magazine, Oct. 18, 1770, pp. 109-111; Scots Magazine, Oct. 1770,
pp. 533-34.

33. London Magazine, Nov. 1770, pp. 581-588.

34. Weekly Magazine, Nov. 15, 1770, p. 213.

35. Ibid., Jan. 24, 1771, p. 114.

36. London Gazette, Oct. 6, 1770.

37. Charles F. Mullett, "A Century of English Quarantine (1709-1825),"
Bulletin of the History of Medicine, vol. 22, no. 6 (Nov.-Dec. 1949), pp. 532-
534.

38. London Gazette, Oct. 20, Nov. 1, Nov. 20, Dec. 1, Dec. 9, 1770.

39. Ibid., May 4, 18, 25, 1771.

40. Ibid., Jan. 29, Feb. 23, May 25, 1771.

41. Weekly Magazine, May 30, 1771, p. 282.

42. Cathcart to Halifax, 19 April 1771, PROSP, 91/87, p. 190v.

43. Arkhiv gosudarstvennogo soveta, vol. 1, pt. 1 (St. Petersburg, 1869),
p. 407.

44. L. F. Hirst, The Conquest of Plague (Oxford, 1953), p. 76.

45. London Magazine, Aug. 1771, p. 424; Weekly Magazine, Sept. 3, 1771,
pp. 311-312; London Magazine, Sept. 1771, p. 474; London Gazette, Sept. 24,
1771; Cathcart to Suffolk, 26 Aug. 1771, PROSP, 91/88, p. 120.

46. Weekly Magazine, Nov. 7, 1771, p. 186.

47. Cathcart to Suffolk, 20 Sept. 1771, SIRIO, vol. 19, pp. 231-234; Arkhiv
gosudarstvennogo soveta, vol. 1, pt. 1, pp. 418-420.

48. William Richardson, Anecdotes of the Russian Empire (London, 1784; reprinted London, 1968), p. 450.

49. Lobkowitz to Kaunitz, 24 Dec. 1771, SIRIO, vol. 109, p. 619.

50. Cathcart to Suffolk, 23 Sept. 1771, PROSP, 91/88, pp. 161v.-162.

51. Cathcart to Suffolk, 18 Nov. and 22 Nov. 1771; British Factory to Cathcart, 22 Nov. 1771, PROSP, 91/88, pp. 259-260, 265.

52. Suffolk to Cathcart, 5 Nov. 1771, PROSP, 91/88, p. 179.

53. Daily Advertiser (London), Oct. 23, 25, 26, 1771; London Gazette,
Nov. 2, 1771.

54. Suffolk to Cathcart and to Swallow, 5 Nov. 1771; Privy Council order of 4
Nov. 1771, PROSP, 91/88, pp. 179-182v., 190-191.

55. Daily Advertiser, Nov. 5, 1771.

56. Ibid., Nov. 7, 1771; London Gazette, Nov. 9, 1771; Suffolk to Cathcart,
8 Nov. 1771; order of the king in council, 8 Nov. 1771, PROSP, 91/88, pp. 194,
196-198v.

57. London Gazette, Jan. 21, 1771.

58. Ibid., Nov. 23, 1771; Daily Advertiser, Nov. 6 and Nov. 12, 1771;
March 31, 1772.

59. Suffolk to Cathcart, 31 Jan. 1772, PROSP, 91/89, pp. 1-3.

60. Swallow to Suffolk, 22 Nov. 1771, PROSP, 91/88, pp. 307-307v.

61. Catherine II, notes to postdirector Ek, Sept. 1771, SIRIO, vol. 13,
pp. 169-171.

62. Swallow to Suffolk, 29 Nov. and 20 Dec. 1771; Cathcart to Suffolk, 30
Dec. 1771, PROSP, 91/88, pp. 291-294v., 320-323v.; 91/89, pp. 21-27.

63. Cathcart to Suffolk, 3 Jan. 1772; Swallow to Suffolk, 7 Feb. 1772,
PROSP, 91/89, pp. 28-29v., 101-102.

64. Suffolk to Cathcart, 20 March 1772; Cathcart to Suffolk, 6 April 1772,
PROSP, 91/89, pp. 116, 184; London Gazette, May 16, 1772; Privy Council Order,
13 May 1772, PROSP, 91/89, pp. 185-185v.; Suffolk to Swallow, 5 June 1772;

Swallow to Suffolk, 10 July 1772; Suffolk to Swallow, 28 Aug. 1772, PROSP,
91/90, pp. 24, 133-135, 158; London Gazette, July 11, 1772.

65. Swallow to Suffolk, 31 July 1772; Eden to Gunning, 11 Sept. 1772,
PROSP, 91/90, pp. 174-174v., 195; London Gazette, Sept. 12, 1772.

66. Matthew Guthrie, "Observations on the Plague, Quarantines, & c. in a
Letter from Dr. Matthew Guthrie, Physician at St. Petersburgh, to Dr. Duncan,"
Medical Commentaries (Edinburgh), vol. 8, pt. 2 (1783), pp. 355-356.

67. Shafonskii, Opisanie morovoi iazvy, p. 131; Daily Advertiser, Dec. 7,
1771; Anthony Cross, "The British in Catherine's Russia: A Preliminary
Survey," in J. G. Garrard, ed., The Eighteenth Century in Russia (Oxford,
1973), pp. 253-254.

68. Matthew Guthrie, reflections on the plague in Moscow in 1771, in "Sup-
plemental Tour of Taurida" (1804-1805), British Museum, Additional Manu-
scripts No. 14388, fols. 195-197. Professor K. A. Papmehl of the University
of Western Ontario, who is preparing an edition of Guthrie's works, gener-
ously furnished me a typescript of these unpublished notes as well as a
copy of the publication cited in note 66.

69. Guthrie, "Observations on the Plague," pp. 346-351, 357.

70. Dr. John Haygarth to John Howard, 19 June 1789, in The Works of John
Howard, Esq., vol. II, Containing the History of Lazarettos; An Account of
the Principal Lazarettos in Europe; with Various Papers Relative to the Plague.
. ., 2d. ed. (London, 1791), sect. III, p. 31.

71. Mullett, The Bubonic Plague and England, pp. 320-322; John T. Alexander,
"Plague in Russia and Danilo Samoilovich: An Historiographical Comment and
Research Note," Canadian-American Slavic Studies, vol. 8, no. 4 (Winter 1974),
p. 527.

Bibliographical Note

Russian medical history in general, and plague epidemics in Russia
in particular, have attracted slight attention from scholars outside
Russia. Hence there is presently little literature of substance about
these subjects in languages other than Russian. The considerable scholarship in Russian, moreover, is not well known to the general run of historians,
inside as well as outside the Soviet Union, and its quality is not consistent.
This situation promises to change in the near future, for several British
and American researchers have begun work on these and related subjects.
Still, compared to the voluminous scholarship on bubonic plague in western
Europe and the British Isles, its Russian manifestations remain little
studied and less known. Thus the present discussion seeks to enumerate
some of the more significant bibliographies, theoretical threatises, primary sources, and historical studies concerning plague epidemics in Russia.

Five works offer extensive bibliographical coverage: A. A. Frari,
Della Peste e della Pubblica Amministrazione Sanitaria, vol. I (Venice,
1840); Georg Sticker, Abhandlungen aus der Seuchengeschichte und Seuchenlehre,
vol. I: Die Pest, pts. 1-2 (Giessen, 1908-1910); D. M. Rossiiskii,
Istoriia vseobshchei i otechestvennoi meditsiny i zdravookhraneniia:
Bibliografiia (996-1954 gg.) (Moscow, 1956); Robert Pollitzer, Plague and
Plague Control in the Soviet Union: History and Bibliography through 1964
(The Institute of Contemporary Russian Studies, Fordham University, Bronx,
New York, 1966); and P. I. Anisimov, T. I. Anisimova, and Z. A. Koneva,
comps., Chuma: Bibliografiia otechestvennoi literatury 1740-1964 gg.
(Saratov, 1968). More recent literature may be found in Current Work in
the History of Medicine: An International Bibliography, published quarterly

by the Wellcome Institute for the History of Medicine in London, and in the monthly Index Medicus issued by the National Library of Medicine in Bethesda, Maryland.

The bionomics and etiology of plague are treated at length in the synthesizing works of L. F. Hirst, The Conquest of Plague: A Study of the Evolution of Epidemiology (Oxford, 1953) and Robert Pollitzer, Plague (Geneva, 1954). These should be supplemented by more recent summaries of research and field work, such as H. H. Mitchell, Plague in the United States: An Assessment of Its Significance as a Problem Following a Thermonuclear War (published by the Rand Corporation for the Technical Analysis Branch of the U.S. Atomic Energy Commission, June, 1966); Jack D. Poland, "Plague," in Paul D. Hoeprich, ed., Infectious Diseases: A Guide to the Understanding and Management of Infectious Processes (New York, 1972), 1141-1148; K. F. Meyer, "Pasteurella and Francisella," in Rene J. Dubois and James G. Hirsch, eds., Bacterial and Mycotic Infections of Man, 4th ed. (Philadelphia and Montreal, 1965), 659-697; and William P. Reed et al., "Bubonic Plague in the Southwestern United States: A Review of Recent Experience," Medicine, vol. 49, no. 6 (November 1970), 465-486.

Numerous primary sources are listed in the bibliographies cited above. For the Moscow epidemic of 1771, the single most important collection of sources is the volume that Dr. A. F. Shafonskii compiled for the plague commission of 1771-75: Opisanie morovoi iazvy, bvyshei v stolichnom gorode Moskve s 1770, po 19772 god, s prilozheniem vsekh dlia prekrashcheniia onoi togda ustanovlennykh uchrezhdenii (Moscow, 1775; St. Petersburg, 1787). Legislation for the period is preserved in Polnoe sobranie zakonov Rossiiskoi imperii, 1st ser. (St. Petersburg, 1830), vol. 19. St. Petersburg's policy may be followed in the protocols of the empress's council, Arkhiv gosudarstvennogo soveta, vol. I, pt. 1 (St. Petersburg, 1869). Catherine II's

general correspondence during the epidemic is printed in <u>Sbornik imperator-</u>
<u>skogo russkogo istoricheskogo obshchestva</u>, vol. 13 (St. Petersburg, 1874).
Her correspondence with P. D. Eropkin is reproduced in Ia. Rost, ed.,
<u>Vysochaishiia sobstvennoruchnyia pis'ma i poveleniia...Imperatritsy Ekateriny</u>
<u>Velikiia, k... Petru Dmitrievichu Erapkinu... i ego doneseniia</u> (Moscow, 1808);
while that with P. S. Saltykov, the governor-general of Moscow, is in
"Pis'ma Imperatritsy Ekateriny Velikoi k fel'dmarshalu grafu Petru Semenovichu
Saltykovu, 1762-1771," <u>Russkii arkhiv</u>, no. 9 (1886), 5-105.

Besides Mertens, several other medical practitioners left accounts of
their experiences during the epidemic and their thoughts about the disease.
Indeed, Mertens' book provoked a lengthy and bitter retort from Danilo
Samoilovich, <u>Mémoire sur la peste, qui, en 1771, ravagea l'Empire de Russie,</u>
<u>sur-tout Moscou, la Capitale</u> (Paris, 1783), which also appeared in German
(Leipzig, 1785), then dropped from sight for almost a century and a half
before being translated into Russian along with several of his other writings:
B. S. Bessmertnyi and O. I. Karakhanian, eds., Danilo Samoilovich, <u>Izbrannye</u>
<u>proizvedeniia</u>, 2 vols. (Moscow, 1949-1952). Samoilovich's criticism of
Mertens met rebuttal from Gustav Orraus, <u>Descriptio pestis, quae anno 1770</u>
<u>in Jassia et 1771 in Moscua grassata est</u> (Petropoli, 1784) and Ivan Vien,
<u>Loimologiia ili opisanie morovoi iazvy, ee sushchestva, proizshestviia,</u>
<u>prichin, porazheniia i proizvodstva pripadkov, s pokazaniem obraza predokh-</u>
<u>raneniia i vrachevaniia seia skorbi</u> (St. Petersburg, 1786).

The best scholarly appraisals of the Moscow epidemic remain the long
article of A. Brikner (Alexander Brückner), "O chume v Moskve 1771 goda,"
<u>Russkii vestnik</u>, vol. 173, no. 9 (Sept. 1884), 5-48; no. 10 (Oct. 1884),
502-568, who first made extensive use of the medical accounts of the epidemic,
and the long chapter of F. A. Derbek, <u>Istoriia chumnykh epidemii v Rossii s</u>

osnovaniia gosudarstva do nastoiashchego vremeni (St. Petersburg, 1905),

whose book is still the only survey of the subject. Unfortunately the

Russian original is less known than a severe abridgement in German: Franz

Dörbeck, Geschichte der Pestepidemien in Russland von der Gründung des

Reiches bis auf die Gegenwart (Breslau, 1906). Brikner's work, by contrast,

is available in a full German edition: A. Brückner, "Die Pest in Moskau,"

Russische Revue, vol. 24 (St. Petersburg, 1884), 301-367, 389-424. Both

these older works outshine the few Soviet treatments, such as P. K. Ale-

firenko, "Chumnyi bunt v Moskve v 1771 godu," Voprosy istorii, no. 4

(April 1947), 82-88; the same author's contribution to S. V. Bakhrushin

et al., eds., Istoriia Moskvy, vol. 2 (Moscow, 1953); and the chapter in

K. G. Vasil'ev and A. E. Segal, Istoriia epidemii v Rossii (Materialy i

ocherki) (Moscow, 1960).

In English there are summaries in Frank G. Clemow, "Plague Epidemics

in Russia: Some Historical Notes," The Indian Medical Gazette (Calcutta),

vol. 33 (Sept.-Oct. 1898), 331-336, 363-368, and Friedrich Prinzing,

Epidemics Resulting from Wars (Oxford, 1916). Some aspects are discussed

by Walther Kirchner, "The Black Death: New Insights into 18th Century

Attitudes toward Bubonic Plague," Clinical Pediatrics, vol. 7, no. 7 (July,

1968), 432-436, who has also published a companion piece in German: "Zur

Geschichte der Pest in Europa: Ihr letztes Auftreten im russischen Heer,"

Saeculum, vol. 20, no. 1 (1969), 82-92. Broader than their titles may indi-

cate are two recent studies by John T. Alexander: "Catherine II, Bubonic

Plague, and the Problem of Industry in Moscow," American Historical Review,

vol. 79, no. 3 (June 1974), 637-671, and "Plague in Russia and Danilo

Samoilovich: An Historiographical Comment and Research Note," Canadian-

American Slavic Studies, vol. 8, no. 4 (Winter 1974), 525-531. The latter exposes the shortcomings of Areta O. Kowal, "Danilo Samoilowitz: An Eighteenth Century Ukrainian Epidemiologist and His Role in the Moscow Plague (1770-72)," Journal of the History of Medicine and Allied Sciences, vol. 27, no. 4 (October 1972), 434-446.

ADDENDA. WRITINGS APPEARING IN 1976 AND 1977

For a recent, massive study of plague in Europe and the Mediterranean that includes some treatment of Russia, see Jean-Noël Biraben, Les hommes et la peste en France et dans les pays européens et méditerranéens, 2 vols. (Paris and La Haye, 1975-76), Ecole des hautes études en sciences sociales, centre de recherches historiques, in the series Civilisation et Sociétés, vols. 35-36, the second volume of which contains a huge bibliography (pp. 186-413). On the Black Death in Russia, see Lawrence N. Langer, "The Black Death in Russia: Its Effects upon Urban Labor," Russian History, vol. 2, no. 1 (1975), 53-67, and the same author's forthcoming (1977) article in Canadian-American Slavic Studies: "Plague and the Russian Countryside: Monastic Estates in the Late Fourteenth and Fifteenth Centuries." An important contribution with implications for Russia is the work of John D. Post, "Famine, Mortality, and Epidemic Disease in the Process of Modernization," Economic History Review, 2nd series, vol. 29, no.1 (1976), 14-37, and his new book, The Last Great Subsistence Crisis in the Western World (Baltimore, 1976). For a global view of epidemic disease that synthesizes much specialized research and devotes much attention to developments within the Eurasian steppe zone, see William H. McNeill, Plagues and Peoples (New York, 1976).

AN

ACCOUNT

OF THE

PLAGUE

WHICH

RAGED AT MOSCOW,

IN

1771.

By CHARLES DE MERTENS, M.D.

MEMBER OF THE MEDICAL COLLEGES OF VIENNA AND
STRASBURG, FORMERLY IMPERIAL AND ROYAL
CENSOR, AND CORRESPONDING MEMBER
OF THE MEDICAL SOCIETY
AT PARIS.

TRANSLATED FROM THE FRENCH, WITH NOTES.

LONDON.

PRINTED FOR F. AND C. RIVINGTON, NO. 62
ST. PAUL'S CHURCH-YARD

1799

PREFACE

HISTORIES of the Plague, exhibiting the modifications it undergoes in different climates, muſt at all times and in all places be acceptable, if not to the public at large, at leaſt to that claſs of perſons who make the art of medicine their ſtudy and employ: But, to a country ſituated like our own, hiſtories of this terrible diſorder occurring in the northern parts of Europe are more particularly intereſting, by holding up to our view a picture of what it probably would be, whenever it ſhould viſit us again. Such a picture is preſented to us in the hiſtory of the plague which depopulated Moſcow and other parts of the Ruſſian empire,

A   in

in the year 1771, and which forms the subject of the following pages. What, at the present time, must give a greater degree of interest to such a subject, is the danger to which we are exposed of importing the pestilential contagion from America *, on the one hand, and from Turkey and the Levant on the other: For, although the cold has, happily, suppressed for the present the pestilence which has been committing such dreadful ravages at Philadelphia and New York; yet is it to be feared that it may be retained in many houses, and lie dormant in various goods, ready to break out again, whenever it shall be favoured by the weather †: And no

---

* Whatever doubts might have been entertained, as to the real nature of the yellow fever, on its first appearance in North America, I believe almost all physicians are now agreed that it is the plague, with such modifications as are easily referable to difference of climate and different mode of living.

† This can hardly fail to be the case until the American government shall have recourse to some of those vigorous measures for eradicating the contagion which are mentioned in the following pages.

one

one who is acquainted with the nature of that contagion can deny the poffibility of its importation from America into this country, either now or hereafter, by infected perfons or infected merchandife. On the other hand, are we not threatened with a fimilar danger from the Eaft? In executing the hoftile operations which are going forwards in the Mediterranean, it feems fcarcely poffible for our fleets and armies to keep clear of contagion. No nation was ever long engaged in a war with the Turks, without taking the plague. In this refpect they are as much to be dreaded by their friends as their foes. If, in the prefent conteft, Italy, and France, and England fhall efcape this fcourge, it will form an exception to paft events, which all Europe muft devoutly pray for.

Under thefe circumftances the Tranflator thought it would be ufeful to call the attention of the practitioners in medicine of this country, to the fubject of peftilential contagion, by publifhing the following Account of the Plague at Mofcow in the year 1771.

Befides

Besides the narrative of the rise and progress of the disorder, and the description of its symptoms and treatment, this account contains also a detail of the methods which were successfully employed in that city for checking and totally extinguishing the contagion; and in particular a detail of the means by which a large edifice, situated in the centre of Moscow, and containing about one thousand four hundred persons, was preserved from the pestilence during the whole of the time that it raged there.

This account is translated from a treatise republished in French, and originally written in Latin by Dr. Mertens, under the following title: "*Traité de la Peste, contenant l'Histoire de celle qui a régné à Moscou en* 1771; *par Charles de Mertens, Docteur en Medecine, &c. ouvrage publié d'abord en Latin* * ; *actuellement mis en François, &c. à Vienne,* 1784." The author (who was physician to the

* In a work, entitled Observationes de Febribus putridis, de Peste, &c. published at Vienna, in 1778.

Foundling

Foundling-Hofpital, at Mofcow, and refided in that city during the whole of the time that the plague raged there) divides his treatife into four chapters; in the firft of which he gives a hiftory of the plague as it appeared at Mofcow; in the fecond, he treats of the diagnofis: in the third, of the curative treatment; and in the fourth, of the precautions or methods of prevention.

So many works have been publifhed on the plague, that whoever writes a regular treatife on this diforder cannot avoid repeating many obfervations that have been made by others before him. Hence, inftead of dividing the prefent pamphlet into chapters and fections, and following the original word for word throughout; the tranflator has taken the liberty of extracting from the two laft chapters thofe parts only which contain new obfervations, or which have an immediate reference to the narrative; which laft he has tranflated entire, excepting half a dozen lines at the beginning, that feem to have been introduced by the author for no other pur-

pofe

pose but that of quoting professor *Schreiber's* *
work on the plague, which broke out in the
Ukraine in the years 1738 and 1739.

Besides the preface †, and some other matters noticed in their respective places, the
following topics of discussion have been
omitted; viz. 1st. *the comparison between the
plague and the smallpox*; 2d. *the reflexions on
the inoculation of the plague*; 3d. *the precautions to be employed in wars with the Turks*;

---

* *Schreiber* Observat. et Cogitat. de Pestilentia quæ
1738 & 1739, in Ukrania grassata est.

† The author's preface or introduction is wholly con-
troversial. It consists of a reply to Mr. *Samoilowoitz*, who
had attempted, in a very illiberal manner, to detract from
the merit of the author's publication. This reply is accompanied with copies of the certificates and testimonials received from the lieutenant of the police, the governours of
the Foundling-Hospital, the lieutenant-general of Moscow,
Count Panin, the privy counsellor de Betzky, &c. relative
to his advice and exertions during the time of the plague.
These vouchers completely refute his adversary's charges;
but as they and the rest of the preface present no facts relative to the history or treatment of the disorder, they cannot be interesting to any but the author's friends, and are
therefore omitted.

and

and 4th. *the precautions continually neceſſary in places expoſed to the peſtilential contagion.*

Theſe topics have been omitted, becauſe with regard to the firſt, as the ſmallpox and the plague agree in no other reſpect but in that of being propagated by contagion, a compariſon between them ſeems to be quite unneceſſary; becauſe, as to the ſecond, the inoculation of the plague is proved to be uſe-leſs by the well-eſtabliſhed fact, that the ſame perſon is ſuſceptible of taking it ſeveral times * ; and becauſe with regard to the third and fourth points, they only lead to repeti-tions of general and particular precautions mentioned in other parts of the pamphlet, or ſuggeſt hints which do not apply to an inſular ſituation like ours.

Next to a detail of all the events which took place during the raging of the plague

---

* Notwithſtanding this, Mr. *Samoilowitz* contends ſtrenuouſly for the inoculation of this diſorder, in a pam-phlet entitled " Memoire ſur l'Inoculation de la Peſte, &c. Straſbourg, 1782."

at Mofcow, the tranflator has efpecially aimed
at a full and accurate delineation of the
fymptoms. In doing this, he has taken the
pains to compare the defcription given by Dr.
Mertens, with thofe of two other writers on
the fame fubject; viz.*Orræus* and *Samoïlowitz*.
Thus he flatters himfelf that all the different types and modifications which the
plague affumes in the Northern parts of
Europe, are here developed in fuch a manner, as to enable thofe who have never feen
the diforder, to detect it on its firft appearance, or in its early progrefs, fhould this
country have the misfortune to be vifited by
it again.

January 2, 1799.

themſelves any further trouble about the means of prevention.

This idea of ſecurity, which was countenanced by the before-mentioned ſtate-phyſician, Dr. *Rinder*, continued until the month of March. The medical conſultations ceaſed. In ſpite of all our efforts to the contrary, every kind of precaution was neglected in the city; it was only at the military-hoſpital that, by order of the Empreſs, the means of prevention were ſtill obſerved; in conſequence whereof the plague was entirely ſuppreſſed there, after twenty-four perſons had been ſeized with it, only two of whom recovered *. Six weeks after the death of the laſt of them, all their clothes, beds, &c. together with the houſe, to which they had been removed, and which was built of wood, were burnt. The hoſpital was opened again at the end of February.

* *Orræus* ſtates, that of the whole number, which conſiſted of thirty, twenty-two died, five recovered, and three eſcaped infection. *Deſcriptio Peſtis*, p. 26. Tranſlator.

The

The generality of mankind judge of things by events only; and will never believe that the plague is among them, until they have certain proof thereof in the number of funerals *. It is owing to this and other mistaken notions, that the plague is not put a stop to in the beginning; at which period it may be compared to a spark which might easily be extinguished, but which, if left to itself, bursts out into a conflagration which nothing can resist.

The opinion which went to assure the inhabitants that they were safe from the plague, was very generally believed, as in such cases almost always happens †. It only remained

---

* We have omitted a sentence or two in this paragragh which threw no light on the subject, and might have appeared exceptionable to some readers. Tr.

† The author relates in a note, which it did not appear necessary to translate entire, that he found himself in a very disagreeable situation, in consequence of having been one of the first to assert the existence of the plague. The language used by some rival practitioners on this occasion, tended (as he believes) to stir up the populace to attack his house in the manner hereafter mentioned.

for

for us to confole ourfelves with the con-
fcioufnefs of having difcharged our duty faith-
fully, and to the beft of our abilities.
Would to God that the bufinefs had ftopped
here, and that what afterwards took place
had not confirmed the truth of our affertions.
We fhould not then have beheld the dreadful deftruction of fo many of our fellow-
creatures, nor have witneffed the moft hor-
rid of all public calamities.

On the 11th of March we are again
convened at the Board of Health. In the
centre of the town there was a large building
ufed for manufacturing clothing for the army ;
three thoufand perfons were employed in it,
nearly a third part of whom, of the moft
neceffitous clafs, occupied the ground-floors ;
the reft, after working there the whole day,
returned in the evening to their refpective
homes, in different parts of the town. Dr.
Yagelfky, at that time fecond phyfician to the
Military Hofpital, whom the Governor-General had fent to the manufactory in the morning, brings word that he had found feveral
patients,

patients, (eight to the beft of my recollec-
tion) labouring under the fame diforder, (accompanied with petechiæ, vibices, carbuncles, and buboes) which he had feen three
months before at the military hofpital ; and
that on feven dead bodies which he had examined, he had perceived fimilar appearances.
On enquiring of the workmen in the manufactory, in what manner, and how long this
diforder had made its appearance among them,
he was told that a woman who had a fwelling in her cheek, had betaken herfelf to
one of her relations who lived in the manufactory, and had died there ; and that, from
that time, one or other of them was every
day taken ill of the diforder. They further ftated, that from the period above-
mentioned to the prefent day, they had loft
one hundred and feventeen perfons, including
the feven dead bodies not yet interred.
This account given by Dr. *Yagelfky,* was cor-
roborated by two other phyficians, who had
been fent the fame day to examine the patients and dead bodies.

In

In a Memoir addreſſed to the Governor-
General and the Senate (by whom we had
been called together) we renew our declara-
tions, that this diſorder is the plague *; and
we adviſe them to remove out of the town
all the perſons dwelling in the manufactory,
taking care to ſeparate the ſick from the
healthy; that they ſhould order the clothes
and furniture of the dead and infected to be
burnt; and that the ſtricteſt ſearch ſhould
be made to find out whether the contagion
exiſted in any other part of the city. The
inhabitants are again ſeized with a panic;
and they now too well perceive the conſe-
quences of their neglect of the precautions
recommended. We were thirteen phyſicians
at this meeting †, two of whom, who three
months before had agreed with us that the
diſeaſe which broke out at the military hoſ-

* See Guſtavi Orræi Deſcriptio Peſtis. 4to. Petro-
poli, 1784, p. 29.

† The ſtate phyſician, Dr. Rinder, was attacked at
the end of February with a gangrenous ulcer in the leg,
which prevented his attendance at this meeting:—He
died ſoon after.

pital

pital was the plague, now said that the present disorder was not the plague, but a putrid fever; an opinion which they enforced in a separate conference with the Senate. These two physicians (Drs. *Kuhlmann* and *Schiadan*) who still differed from us in opinion, had been led into their error, by observing that the number of deaths in the town was not greater than usual, but rather less than in the preceding years, and that there were very few people ill.

Some days after, being summoned to meet the other physicians and surgeons at the senate, where each of us was required to deliver our sentiments explicitly, I affirmed, in the most solemn manner, that I was thoroughly convinced that the disease under consideration was the plague; ten of my colleagues were of the same opinion, and the two others before mentioned still maintained the contrary *; nevertheless, they admitted the propriety of adopting precautions against

* Orræus, as before quoted, p. 29.

a disa diforder, which, though not the plague, was of a contagious nature.

The firft day (the 11th of March) is fpent in deliberations. The infected building is fhut up, and guards are placed there, to prevent any perfon from going in or coming out. Several make their efcape through the windows, and the reft are removed out of the town during the night, the uninfected to the convent of St. Simon, and the infected to the convent of St. Nicholas, one of which is diftant fix, and the other eight verfts *; from Mofcow. Thefe convents are furrounded with high walls, and have only one entrance. As it was difcovered that fome had died among the workmen who lived in their own houfes, thefe were taken to a third convent, fituated in like manner out of the town. Orders were given to the furgeons who had the care of all thefe people, to tranfmit daily to the Board of Health a lift of the fick and dead. A committee of phyficians

---

* Three verfts are equal to two Englifh miles. Tr.

was

was appointed to regulate every thing concerning the treatment of the fick, and the
keeping of thofe who were performing quarantine free from infection; and great attention was paid to the interment of the dead.
Drs. *Erafmus* and *Yagelfky* (now no more!)
were entitled to great praife for the manner
in which they acquitted themfelves in this
bufinefs. When any one of thofe who were
under quarantine was taken ill, he was put
in a feparate room, and kept there until the
fymptoms of the plague fhewed themfelves,
when he was conveyed in a carriage, by perfons hired for that purpofe, to the peft-
houfe, viz. the convent of St. Nicholas.

The public baths, where the people are
accuftomed to go, at leaft once a week,
were fhut up. The town was divided into
feven diftricts, to each of which one phyfician and two furgeons were appointed, for
the purpofe of examining all the fick as well
as the dead bodies; in which bufinefs police-
officers were joined with them. It was for-
bidden to bury the dead within the city; proper

per places for burying-grounds were fixed upon at fome diftance from the town. It was ordered, that whenever any one of the common people fhould be feized with the plague, he fhould be fent to the hofpital of St. Nicholas, and that, after burning his clothes and furniture, thofe who had been living in the fame apartment fhould be detained for the fpace of forty days in fome buildings appropriated to that purpofe out of the town; that if the like occurrence fhould happen in the houfe of a principal inhabitant or perfon of rank, all the fervants who had been in the fame room with the patient fhould perform quarantine, and that the mafter, together with all his family, fhould remain fhut up in his own houfe for the fpace of eleven days. All this was fanctioned and paffed into the form of a law by a refolution of the Senate. General *Peter Demitrewich de Yeropkin,* not more diftinguifhed by his birth and valour than by his polifhed manners and humane difpofition, was appointed by the Emprefs, Director-General of Health.

Notwithſtanding what had happened, the number of thoſe who were convinced that the plague had reached Moſcow, was as yet inconſiderable. Dr. *Orræus*, phyſician to the army, who had viſited impeſted patients at Jaſſy, was now paſſing through Moſcow in his way to Peterſburgh, and was requeſted to examine the ſick and dead bodies before mentioned, which he accordingly did, and declared, that the diſorder was exactly like that which, a ſhort time before, had proved ſo deſtructive in Moldavia and Wallachia; that it was, in fact, the plague. This was further confirmed by Dr. *Lærch*, who was juſt returned from Kiow, where he had remained during the time that the plague raged there.

The weather continued very cold until the middle of April, in conſequence of which the contagion became more fixed and inactive, attacking only thoſe who dwelt with the infected. In the peſt-houſe, the daily number of deaths did not exceed three or four; and of the manufacturers who were performing
quarantine

quarantine only about the same number fell ill.

According to the reports of the physicians, surgeons, and police-officers, the town appeared to be healthy. Almost every body believed that the physicians who had called the disorder the plague, had imposed upon the public; others entertained doubts on the subject. Things went on in this way until the middle of June, during which time nearly two hundred persons had died at the hospital of St. Nicholas. The number of sick and dead diminished daily there, in so much that, for a whole week, although the weather was very warm, not one fell ill of the disorder, and there only remained in the hospital a few convalescents. No further vestige of the disorder could be traced in the town.

As among the workmen of the manufactory, who had been removed from their own houses to a third convent at a distance from the other two, in order to perform quaran-

C 2   tine,

tine, not one had been attacked with the diforder for the space of two months, they were allowed to return to their respective homes.

We now began to flatter ourselves that the plague had been entirely eradicated by the precautions which had been adopted. Scarcely, however, had we indulged in these fond hopes, when, towards the end of June, some people are taken ill of the same diforder at the hospital of St. Simon, where the quarantine was performed. On the 2d of July, six people die in one night at a house in the suburb of Preobraginsky; a seventh, who lived with them, absconded *. Livid spots, buboes, and carbuncles are found upon the dead bodies. On the following days, many of the common people fall sick in different quarters of the town, and the mor-

* In what manner the contagion got among these people could not be ascertained. Perhaps, through the negligence of the centinels, they had some communication with the persons under quarantine; or had become infected by bringing into use clothes and other effects, which the laft-mentioned persons might have concealed under ground before their removal to the quarantine-hospital.

tality

tality increafes to fuch a pitch, that the number of deaths, which commonly amounted to about ten or fifteen *per* day, and which, even during the prevalence of putrid fevers (as was the cafe for the two laft years) did not exceed thirty, amounted at the end of July to as many as two hundred in the fpace of twenty-four hours. The fick, as well as the dead bodies, exhibited large purple fpots and vibices; in many there were carbuncles and buboes. Some died fuddenly, or in the fpace of twenty-four hours, before the buboes and carbuncles had time to come out; but the greateft number died on the third or fourth day.

In the middle of Auguft, the number of deaths amounted daily to four hundred; and at the end of the fame month to as many as fix hundred. At this time buboes and carbuncles were more frequent than they had been in July. At the beginning of September there were feven hundred deaths in the fpace of twenty-four hours; in a few days, there were eight hundred deaths with-

in

in the same number of hours; and a short time after, the deaths amounted to one thousand in a day!

The havoc was still greater during the time of the riots, which began on the 15th of September, in the evening; when an outrageous mob broke open the pest-houses and quarantine-hospitals, renewing all the religious ceremonies which it is customary with them to perform at the bed-side of the sick *, and digging up the dead bodies and burying them afresh in the city. Agreeably to their ancient custom, the people began again to embrace the dead, despising all manner of precaution, which they declared to be of no avail, as the public calamity (I repeat their own words) was sent by God, to punish them for having neglected their ancient forms of worship. They further insisted, that as it was pre-ordained who should

* Besides praying by them in the ordinary manner, it is customary, in Russia, to carry in great pomp to the sick the images of their saints, which every person present kisses in rotation.

and

and who fhould not die, they muft await their deftiny; therefore, that all endeavours to avoid the contagion were only a trouble to themfelves, and an infult to the Divinity, whofe wrath was only to be appeafed by their refufing all human affiftance *. *General Yeropkin*, with a fmall party of foldiers drawn together as fpeedily as poffible, difperfed the mob, and reftored tranquillity in a few days, after which every thing was placed on its former footing. This vaft concourfe and intermixture of the healthy and infected, caufed the contagion to fpread to fuch a degree, that at this time the daily number of deaths amounted to one thoufand two hundred and upwards!

---

* In their paroxyfm of phrenfy, the populace attempted to wreak their vengeance upon thofe who had laboured for their prefervation. After they had facrificed one victim to their blind rage, they fought for the phyficians and furgeons. Some of the loweft rabble broke into my houfe, and deftroyed every thing they could lay hold of; they alfo went in fearch of the other phyficians and furgeons, and purfued fuch as they met with. Providence refcued us all from their hands. Little fufpecting what was to happen, I had gone four days before, by order of council, to the Foundling-Hofpital, to fuperintend more clofely the health of the children there.

Mofcow,

Moscow, one of the largest cities in
Europe, consists of four circles, or inclo-
sures, one within another; the smallest,
which occupies the centre, is called Krem-
mel; and the second, which surrounds it,
Kitaya, (or Chinese-Town); they are both
inclosed by brick-walls, and the houses
within them are built of brick; the third,
which is called Bielogorod (or White-Town)
is without walls, they having been levelled
with the ground; and, lastly, the fourth
called Zemlanoïgorod (from Zemla, land
or earth, and Gorod, town) is defended by a
ditch and rampart of earth *. In the two
last-named parts of Moscow the houses are,
for the most part, constructed of wood.
These houses do not stand close together,
but are detached with spaces between, and,
in general, only one family inhabits each;
hence they rarely consist of more than one

---

* There is some little variation between this author's
spelling of these Russian names and Mr. *Coxe's*. The last-
mentioned traveller writes the 1st. Kremlin; the 2d. Khi-
taigorod; the 3d. Bielgorod; and the 4th. Semlainogorod.
This last takes its name from the rampart of earth with
which it is surrounded.   Tr.

story,

ſtory, and often of a ground-floor only. The nobles keep a great number of ſervants; and the common people live crouded together in ſmall wooden houſes *.

In winter time the nobles repair to Moſcow, from all parts of the empire, bringing with them a large train of attendants. Great numbers of the common people, who were engaged during the ſummer in agricultural labour, return to this great city in the winter, to gain ſubſiſtence by different employments. This conflux of people makes the town ſo full, from the month of December to March, that the population, at this ſeaſon, amounts, according to ſome computations, to two hundred and fifty thouſand; according to others, to three hundred thouſand. In the month of March, people begin to go into the country again; hence, during the ſummer,

* Mr. *Coxe* deſcribes the wooden houſes of the common people in Moſcow, as mean hovels, in no degree ſuperior to peaſants cottages. It is eaſy to conceive how favourable theſe low and crouded habitations muſt have been to the harbouring and ſpreading of contagion. Tr.

the

the number of inhabitants is, at least, one-fourth less than in winter. In 1771 the fear of catching the plague had caused a much greater number to leave the city; so that I do not think that, in the month of August, there were more than one hundred and fifty thousand remaining in the place. An idea may be formed of the destructive nature of this disorder, and the terrible activity of its poison, by reflecting, that of these one hundred and fifty thousand inhabitants, twelve hundred were daily carried off by it, (in the month of September!) The number of deaths kept at this rate for some days, and then diminished to one thousand. As the populace, during the riots, had re-established all the religious ceremonies customary on burying the dead, almost all their priests, deacons, and other ecclesiastics, fell victims to the contagion.

The people, brought to a sense of their duty, partly by the rigorous measures employed against them, and partly by seeing that the public calamity had been aggravated

by

by their diforderly proceedings, now began
to implore our affiftance. The monafteries
and other peft-houfes were full; the fick
were no longer carried thither; the contagion had fpread every where; infomuch that
the city itfelf might be confidered as one
entire hofpital. All, therefore, we could now
do, was to exhort every individual to take
care of himfelf; to warn all thofe who were
yet free from the contagion, to avoid, as
much as poffible, touching with their bare
hands any infected perfon; to direct them to
burn the clothes, and every thing elfe that
had been ufed by thofe who had been ill of
the plague; and, laftly, to keep their rooms
clean and well aired.

At this time *Count Gregory Orlow* * arrived
at Mofcow, invefted with full powers by the
emprefs. I received an order, in common
with the other phyficians, to deliver, in
writing, my private fentiments on the fubject; we were required to turn our attention
principally to the moft proper meafures for

* Now Prince *Orlow.*

deftroy-destroying the contagion *. Having taken the necessary steps to prevent all further popular commotions, the Count selected, from all our papers, what appeared of most moment, and drew up a set of regulations, as well for the treatment of the sick, as for the keeping of those who were yet well, free from infection. He also ordered new hospitals to be immediately built for the reception of the poor seized with the plague †.

Some months had elapsed since the plague had been carried to many of the villages, as well in the vicinity as at a distance from Moscow. Persons who fled from this city had also carried it with them to Kalomna (Kaluga, according to *Orrœus*), Yaroslaw, and Tula. Inspectors of health, attended

---

* See Addenda, Note B.

† In Russia it is no uncommon thing to have a large edifice built of wood in a few days. See *Coxe's* Travels. To persons unacquainted with this fact, the erecting of new hospitals might seem a very tardy measure for checking the progress of the plague. Tr.

by

by phyficians and furgeons, were fent to thefe infected towns and villages.

A Council of Health was formed, compofed of *General Yeropkin* (who was prefident), of fome counfellors of ftate, and of three phyficians, and one furgeon. This council received daily reports from the phyficians and police-officers, and took cognizance of every thing which related to the health of the inhabitants. Two phyficians, Drs. *Pogaretfky* and *Meltzer*, being offered a reward of one thoufand roubles, undertook, each of them, the care of a pefthofpital; and went thither accordingly.

On the 10th of October the froft fet in; from that day the diforder was lefs fatal, and the contagion became more fixed. The number of fick and dead gradually diminifhed; and the diforder, which a fhort time before had terminated on the fecond or third day, now kept on to the fifth or fixth. Neither thofe large purple fpots, which we have before defcribed, nor carbuncles, were

by

by any means so frequent as they had been; buboes were now almost the only tumours found upon the infected.

The hard frost * which prevailed during the two last months of the year, weakened the pestilential virus to such a degree, that those who attended the sick and buried the dead were in much less danger of being infected; and when they were infected, the symptoms were much milder; so that at this period, several persons who had the plague were but slightly indisposed, and walked about though they had buboes upon them.

At the close of the year 1771, this dreadful scourge ceased, by the blessing of God, at Moscow, and in every other part of the Russian empire. Besides the three towns before-mentioned, upwards of four hundred villages had been infected.

* *Reaumur's* thermometer was constantly in the morning between 16 and 22 degrees below the freezing point.

The

The weather was intenfely cold during the whole of the winter. In order to deftroy all remains of the contagion, the doors and windows of the rooms in which there had been any perfons ill of the plague, were broken and the rooms were fumigated with the antipeftilential powder *; the old wooden houfes were entirely demolifhed. The effects of the plague were traced in every part of the city. Even as late as the month of February, 1772, upwards of four hundred dead bodies were difcovered, which had been fecretly buried the year before in private houfes. So powerful is cold in deftroying the contagion, that not one of thofe who were employed in digging up thefe bodies, and carrying them to the public burying-grounds, became infected †.

* See Addenda, note C.

† Dr. *Pogaretfky*, who had the care of the peft-hofpital, Laforte, told me that fome of the bearers of the dead had put on fheep-fkins that had been worn by the impefted, after having expofed them to the open air for forty-eight hours, in the month of December, when the froft was very intenfe; and that none of them became infected.

The

The total number of perfons carried off by the plague amounted, according to the reports tranfmitted to the Senate and Council of Health, to upwards of feventy thoufand ; more than twenty-two thoufand of this number of deaths happened in the month of Sep-tember alone *. If we add to thefe, the pri-vate and clandeftine interments †, the whole number of deaths in Mofcow will amount to eighty thoufand ‡ : and reckoning thofe who

died

* The author remarks in a note, that the number of deaths in the month of September, probably amounted to as many as twenty-feven thoufand. At this time, which was during the riots, the number of deaths could not be accurately regiftered.

† The number of thefe was by no means inconfidera-ble; for during the height of the plague, there was fcarcely a fufficient number of men, horfes, and carts to carry off the dead; many remained uninterred for two or three days, and were at length taken away by their rela-tions, friends, or poor people hired for that purpofe. Many of thefe could not be regiftered, befides numbers of others who were buried in fecret, and whofe illnefs was never reported to the Senate.

‡ According to the returns made to the Council of Health, and publifhed by *Orræus* (Defcriptio Peftis, p. 48,) the number of perfons carried off by the plague at Mofcow

died in upwards of four hundred villages, and in the three towns of Tula, Yaroslaw and Kalomna (or Kaluga) *, it will follow that this plague swept off altogether as many as an hundred thousand persons!

For carrying away and burying the dead, criminals capitally convicted or condemned to hard labour, were at first employed; but afterwards, when these were not sufficient for the purpose, the poor were hired to per-

cow in the year 1771, did not amount to more than fifty-six thousand seven hundred and seventy-two. It is to be remarked, however, that this list of deaths is dated only from the month of April, whereas the plague broke out in the cloth-manufactory in the beginning of March. Indeed, *Orræus* himself acknowledges, (p. 49,) that a much greater number than what appears from the reports laid before the Council must have died of the plague, as, on pulling down the houses in different parts of the city, so many dead bodies were found that had been secretly interred, and as, moreover, in the beginning of the disorder, the returns were very inaccurately made. Tr.

* These towns did not suffer greatly from the plague, as the inhabitants took warning from the unhappy fate of Moscow, and attended to the necessary precautions from the beginning. It was more destructive in the villages, and particularly in those that were at the greatest distance from Moscow.

form

form this service. Each was provided with a
cloke, gloves, and a mask made of oiled cloth;
and they were cautioned never to touch a
dead body with their bare hands. But they
would not attend to thefe precautions, be-
lieving it to be impoffible . to be hurt by
merely touching the bodies or clothes of the
dead, and attributing the effects of the contagion to an inevitable deftiny. We loft
thoufands of thefe people, who feldom remained well beyond a week. I was informed
by the Infpectors of Health, that moft of
them fell ill about the fourth or fifth day.

The plague, as is generally the cafe, raged
chiefly among the common people; the nobles and better fort of inhabitants efcaped the
contagion, a few only excepted, who fell
victims to their rafhnefs and negligence.
The contagion was communicated folely by
contact of the fick or infected goods; it was
not propagated by the atmofphere, which
appeared in no refpect vitiated during the
whole of the time. When we vifited any

of

of the sick we * went so near them that frequently there was not more than a foot's distance between them and us; and although we used no other precaution but that of not touching their bodies, clothes, or beds, we escaped infection. When I looked at a patient's tongue, I used to hold before my mouth and nose a pocket - handkerchief moistened with vinegar †.

Amid so great a number of deaths, I think there were only three persons of family, a

* I mean those physicians who, with myself, remained in the town; but not such as had the care of the pest-hospitals.

† Although the atmosphere may not be capable of communicating the pestilential contagion beyond a very limited distance from its source, yet to appproach so near as within a foot of the infected, appears to us (notwithstanding the present instance to the contrary) to be a practice not generally safe. Dr. *Russel* proceeded with more caution in his examinations of the infected at Aleppo. He prescribed to most of his patients out of a window, about fifteen feet above them. A stair passed near one of the windows, by which he had such of the infected, whose eruptions he wanted to examine, brought within a smaller distance, viz. within four or five feet. *Russell*, on the Plague, book I. ch. vi. Tr.

few

few of the principal citizens, and not more than three hundred foreigners of the common clafs, who fell victims to the plague; the reft confifted of the loweft order of the Ruf-fian inhabitants. The former only purchafed what was abfolutely neceffary for their fup-port, during the time of the peftilence; whereas the latter bought up every thing which was refcued from the flames, and which of courfe was fold at a very low price; they refufed to burn the goods which came to them by inheritance; and, moreover, car-ried away many things clandeftinely, in fpite of all we could fay or do to the contrary.

Two furgeons died of the plague in the town; and a great number of furgeons-mates and pupils in the hofpitals. Dr. *Poga-retzky* and Mr. *Samoïlowitz*, firft furgeon to the hofpital of St. Nicholas, both caught the infection feveral times; and were cured by critical fweats coming on at the beginning of each attack of the diforder.

The

The foundling hospital, which contained about a thousand children * and four hundred adults (including nurses, servants, masters, and workmen) was kept free from infection by the precautions hereafter mentioned †. Only four workmen, and as many soldiers, who had got over the fences in the night time, were seized at different times; but by immediately separating them from the rest of the house, the disorder was prevented from spreading any farther. Thus this building was kept free from the plague, at the time that it raged in all the other houses around it; a proof that the atmosphere, not only during the frost, but even during the great heat of the summer ‡, did not serve

as

* Almost all the youngest children were out at nurse in the country.

(Mr. *Coxe* relates, that, at the time he was at Moscow, this noble institution contained three thousand foundlings. Tr.)

† See Addenda, D.

‡ It is remarkable, that it is towards the summer-solstice, according to *Russel* (Natural History of Aleppo)

and

as a vehicle for spreading the contagion, which was only propagated by contact of the sick or infected goods *.

The young and robust were more liable to become infected than elderly and infirm persons; pregnant women and nurses were not secure from its attacks. Children under

and *Prosper Alpinus* (Medicina Ægyptiorum) that the plague generally ceases in Asia and Africa; whilst in Europe it rages with the greatest fury at that season, and is only subdued by the winter-cold.

* From the author's expressions in this place, the reader might be led to believe that he meant to restrict the communication of infection to contact of the sick and infected goods; but in other parts of his book, he admits the possibility of the contagion being communicated by the breath and other effluvia from the sick. Indeed there can be no doubt that the pestilential particles are (especially in the worst forms of the disease) contained in the moisture perspired through the skin, and in the vapour emitted from the lungs. If not, where was the use of the precaution, which the author adopted in his own person, of holding a handkerchief moistened with vinegar before the mouth and nose on approaching the sick? The conclusion, from all this is, that the sphere of contagion in cases of the plague, extends to a greater distance (several feet at least) than Dr. *Mertens* imagines. Tr.

four

four years of age were much less readily
infected, but when they were, they exhibited
the worst symptoms.

All who were attacked with the plague
had more or less fever; though in some it
was so slight as to be scarcely perceivable.   In
a few instances, the patients were seized,
from the first, with a furious delirium, accompanied with a high degree of fever; but
the greater part were affected with debility,
and only complained of oppression about the
præcordia, and head-ach *.

After taking great pains to ascertain in
what manner the plague was introduced into
the military hospital, the physician to that
institution at length found out that two soldiers had died there in the month of November, 1770, a short time after their arrival
from Choczim, where the plague was then
raging; and that a Colonel, in whose train

* For a more particular account of the symptoms, see
Addenda, A.

they

they were, had died upon the road. It would feem that the anatomical diffector opened the bodies of thefe foldiers; and that he caught the plague of them. The perfons who waited upon the fick, either became infected by touching the bodies of thefe foldiers whilft they were living; or by handling their clothes, or their bodies after death. Thefe attendants afterwards fpread the contagion among their families.

Thus have we traced the hiftory of the plague which depopulated Mofcow in the year 1771, from its firft appearance to its final extinction. A plain and faithful ftatement of facts, even at the rifk of being tedious, is what has been aimed at in this narrative; for let it be obferved, that it is from fimple details of the origin and progrefs of the plague, as it appears in different places, and of the fymptoms and other circumftances with which it is accompanied, and not from the laboured differtations that have been written upon it by fome voluminous authors, that we can hope to acquire an accurate knowledge of the nature of this diforder, to afcertain the manner in which its contagion is propagated, and laftly to difcover the beft methods of prevention and cure.

ADDENDA.

A.

Symptoms more particularly described.

THE symptoms of the plague vary according to the different conſtitutions of
the perſons whom it attacks, and the ſeaſon
of the year in which it appears. Sometimes it wears the maſk of other diſeaſes;
but in general it is uſhered in by head-ach,
ſtupor, reſembling intoxication, ſhiverings,
depreſſion of ſpirits, and loſs of ſtrength;
theſe are followed by ſome degree of fever,
together with nauſea and vomiting. The
eyes become red, the countenance melancholy, and the tongue white and foul. In
this ſtate of things, the patients are ſometimes capable of ſitting up, and going about
for ſome hours, or even a day or two. They
feel an itching or pain in thoſe parts of the
body

body where buboes and carbuncles are about to appear. During the height of the plague, many of the infected die on the second or third day, before thefe tumours have time to come out, and with no other external marks except petechiæ or purple fpots, which appear a fhort time before death; in fome thefe fpots are altogether wanting. The buboes and carbuncles generally come out on the fecond or third day, feldom on the fourth.

In fome inftances, the plague appears under the form of an inflammatory diforder, being accompanied with great heat, thirft, high-coloured urine, flufhed cheeks, and violent delirium or phrenfy; but in the greater number of cafes it affumes the type of a nervous fever, being accompanied with little heat and thirft, and pale and turbid urine; the patients think themfelves only flightly indifpofed, until a fudden proftration of ftrength, and the eruption of buboes, carbuncles, petechiæ or vibices, announce to themfelves, as well as to thofe who are about them, the danger they are in. In fome few
inftances,

inftances, the plague appears under the form
of an intermittent fever.—Almoft all thofe
who are carried off by this diforder, die before the fixth day; thofe who get over
the feventh day have a good chance of recovery *.

The diverfity of fymptoms above-noticed,
has given rife to the opinion that there are
three different fpecies of the plague, viz. one
which is accompained with petechiæ, another with carbuncles, and a third with buboes; but the hiftory which we have given,
clearly proves, that thefe are only fhades or
modifications of one and the fame diforder,
which is more or lefs violent under different
circumftances and at different feafons. Petechiæ, buboes, and carbuncles often appear
at the fame time in the fame patient, or oc-

* The author did not venture to feel the pulfe of thofe
impefted patients who were under his own care, left he
fhould take infection. As the obfervations communicated
to him by others on this head, which he has inferted in
his book, coincide with thofe of *Orræus* and *Samöilowitz*,
which we fhall afterwards notice, we have omitted them,
to avoid repetition. Tr.

cur

cur in fucceffion. In the month of July,
great numbers of the impefted died before
the tumours came out, having petechiæ only;
whereas in Auguft and September, almoft
every patient had petechiæ, joined with buboes and carbuncles. After the middle of
October, when the contagion was lefs virulent, although it ftill produced petechiæ and
carbuncles, yet they were neither fo malignant nor fo frequent. Before this period,
fcarcely four patients in a hundred recovered;
whereas during the latter months of the year,
the proportion of recoveries was much
greater. *Sydenham* has made the fame obfervation refpecting the plague at London *.
Nature endeavours to throw off the poifon by
buboes. Carbuncles and petechiæ are not

* It will be fufficient for readers in this country to refer
to *Sydenham*'s works, Sect. II. Cap. II. without tranfcribing
the quotation which the author has introduced in this place.
Sydenham obferves of the London plague (1665), that it
was moft fuddenly mortal in the beginning; whereas the
Ruffian plague was the moft rapid in its action when it
was at its height. Dr. *Mertens* reconciles this contrariety
of obfervation, by remarking that the London plague
began in the fummer, a feafon the moft favourable for its
activity. Tr.

critical

critical eruptions; they only denote a putrid condition of the humours, and a great degree of acrimony; whence it follows, that in proportion as buboes are more common, and petechiæ and carbuncles more rare, the milder the plague is *.

———

To this account which Dr. *Mertens* has given of the symptoms which the plague at Moscow exhibited, we shall add the descriptions drawn up by two other practitioners (*Orræus* and *Samoïlowitz*,) who had great opportunities of observation, and who have been more particular in noticing some of the phenomena than our author.

According to *Orræus* (Descriptio Pestis, &c.) the plague in Russia appeared under four different forms or varieties. Of these, he terms the first, *the period of infection;*

* The description and treatment of the buboes, carbuncles, and other eruptions, which are to be found in every treatise on the Plague, the translator has purposely omitted, that the pamphlet might not be swelled out to an unnecessary bulk.

the second, *the flow type*; the third, *the acute type*; and the fourth, *the exceedingly acute type*.

1. In *the period of infection* (which is commonly the forerunner of the other forms of the plague) the contagion, lefs active and virulent, keeps lurking in the body, and produces the following fymptoms, viz. fharp, flying pains in the glandular parts (fuch as the armpit and groins) and in the mufcles of the neck and breaft; ardor urinæ; drowfinefs; an increafed fecretion of the febaceous humour, fo that the fkin is in many parts, and more efpecially in the hands and face, much more unctuous and gloffy than ufual; the belly is coftive, but when moved, there comes away a great quantity of pulpy flimy fæces; the patients complain of a heavinefs of the body (fome compare their limbs to a mafs of lead), great laffitude and faintings. A fwelling, but without much pain, of fome gland (in the groin or armpit) together with dark-red or brown fpots, denote a
higher

higher degree of infection: and a bad taste in the mouth, a viscidity of the saliva, loss of appetite, whiteness and foulness of the tongue, and head-ach, show that the patient is going to be attacked with the plague under one or other of the following types. The above-mentioned symptoms, which continue for a longer or shorter time (in some instances for several days or even weeks) are not accompanied with fever.

2. After the period of infection above described has continued for some time without yielding to medicine, it generally ends in *the flow type of the plague*, which is characterized by the following symptoms; viz. shiverings, followed by a moderate degree of heat (A), a febrile (B), unequal, for the most part weak, and often intermitting pulse; a constant dull

(A) Frequently in the progress of the disease there is no heat on the surface of the body; but the burning heat under the axillæ shows that the internal heat is very intense.

(B) A febrile, but not very quick pulse; sometimes almost natural.

pain in the head (rather, according to the ex-
preſſion of ſome patients, a heavineſs, as if
the head was full of lead); urine pale and
turbid, but without ſediment; tongue foul
and moiſt; very little thirſt; depreſſion of
ſpirits; belly coſtive during the firſt three or
four days, with inflation of the hypo-
chondria and borborygmi, but the abdomen
feels ſoft on preſſure; there is frequent nauſea and vomiting of a ſlimy greeniſh-yellow
ſaburra (c); petechiæ and other eruptions (D)
make their appearance, in ſome ſooner in others

(c) The ſaburra brought up by vomiting, is commonly
of a dirty yellow colour, viſcid, and ſometimes frothy.
The quantity thrown up is aſtoniſhingly great, much
greater than is obſerved in any other fever.

(D) The petechiæ and other eruptions vary in ſize and
colour. They are moſtly ſmall and diſtinct, but ſometimes run together and form broad maculæ, which now
and then end in carbuncles. Their colour in many inſtances is livid or black, in others (when the diſeaſe is
milder) purpliſh, in ſome reddiſh. In convaleſcents, they
turn firſt red, then yellow, and afterwards diſappear.
They are ſo common in the beginning of the plague, that
ſcarcely any one dies without them; though buboes and
carbuncles are not obſervable. Hence thoſe who have
never ſeen the plague under all its forms are apt to be
deceived reſpecting the nature of the diſorder.

later;

later; but in fome they are altogether wanting. The rudiments or germs of buboes
and carbuncles, which were forming during
the period of infection, now gradually increafe in fize, but without being accompanied with violent pain; and new ones arife
in other places; which, if they fuppurate on
the fifth, fixth, or feventh day, fave the life
of the patient: on the other hand, if no
fuppuration takes place, and great debility,
diarrhœa, and delirium come on, the difeafe
terminates fatally, not, however, in fome
cafes till after the fourteenth day.

3. In *the acute type*, the plague is preceded
by a much fhorter indifpofition, fometimes
by none at all, fuddenly feizing perfons in
health. It is characterized by the following
fymptoms: a bitter tafte in the mouth, and
a vifcidity of the faliva; violent head-ach (E);

(E) The patients complain of this more than of any
other fymptom. The pain begins in the frontal finus,
and the orbits of the eyes, and afterwards extends to the
temples and fides of the head as far as to the back part, and
gradually over the whole head; fo, however, as to be
moft violent in the fore part.

rednefs

rednefs of the eyes (F) and face; a very foul,
and fometimes dry tongue; chillinefs fuc-
ceeded by confiderable heat; a much fuller,
ftronger, and quicker pulfe than in the flow
type of the diforder, as well as more thirft,
and deeper coloured urine; coftivenefs; buboes, and carbuncles come out foon after the
attack of fever, or at the fame time with it;
after thefe, others come out; frequent vomitings
fupervene, and a delirium, which is generally
of the low kind (G). If, between the firft
and

(F) The appearance of the eyes in the plague is fuch as,
when once feen, will ever afterwards enable even the com-
moneft obfervers to recognife the difeafe. The eyes are
unufually prominent, and the veffels of the tunica albu-
ginea are turgid with blood, fo as to produce a præterna-
tural rednefs. They are, moreover, watery, fometimes
full of tears (lacrymantes), and have a fparkling fierce-
nefs. But in the advanced ftage of the difeafe, when the
powers of life become exhaufted, the eyes fink in, the
rednefs gradually goes off, and a little while before death
they become dull, and appear as if they had a film over
them.

(G) Although the delirium is rather higher than it is
in the flow type of the plague, yet it is very rarely of the
furious kind, in the prefent type of the difeafe. The patients are affected with ftupor, and lie motionlefs in a

dozing

and fourth day of the attack, the buboes are
refolved (H), or they, as well as the carbuncles, come to fuppuration, the patient recovers: on the other hand, if no fuppuration takes place within that period; if the
buboes and carbuncles increafe to a great fize,
and the delirium continues, then the powers
of life become exhaufted, the pulfe finks,
and death is ufhered in by hæmorrhages, and
a copious exfpuition of thin phlegm (I).

Death

---

dozing ftate; or if they awake, they are perpetually
ftretching out their hands and trying to raife themfelves
up, as if they wanted to get out of bed. They talk in-
ceffantly, but in confequence of the turgid and fwollen
ftate of the tongue, their fpeech is broken and ftuttering
like that of drunken people, fo as to be fcarcely intelli-
gible.

(H) The buboes are difperfed or refolved by critical
fweats breaking out on the firft day of the attack. Often,
at the fame time, there is a difcharge from the urethra of
a white, vifcid fluid, refembling pus, fimilar to what happens in a gleet; but this running is not accompanied with
pain, and ceafes fpontaneoufly after a few days.

(I) A moderate bleeding from the nofe in the beginning of the difeafe, was, efpecially in plethoric habits,
fometimes falutary; but in moft inftances it was other-
wife.

Death takes place on the third, fourth, or fifth day; and it often happens, while the corpfe is yet warm, that petechiæ and other fpots come out. The bodies, after death, appear remarkably pale, foft, fomewhat tumid, flexible, and free from fætor.

4. The plague, *in its moſt acute type*, attacks in various ways; but in relation to the leading fymptoms, it may be reduced to two forms : in the firft, a perfon in perfect health, without any previous marks of infection, is fuddenly feized with a fhort but violent fhivering fit, followed by a hot fit, which al-

wife. Such as fpat up frothy blood, mixed with a great quantity of thin phlegm, though they might not at the time exhibit fymptoms of great debility, or appear to be in danger, did, neverthelefs, contrary to expectation, die foon afterwards. Hæmorrhages happened more frequently, and proved more fatal to women than to men. An immoderate flow of the menfes coming on fuddenly and before the ftated time, carried off the patient in many inftances. When pregnant women were attacked with this type of the plague, they almoft always mifcarried, and loft their lives by the fubfequent hæmorrhage. This was alfo very generally the cafe with thofe who were delivered after having gone their natural time.

ternate

ternate with each other several times; but
the external heat soon goes off, and the skin
feels cool. The pulse is hard and very
quick, with a most violent head-ach and intolerable anxiety about the præcordia (κ);
a furious delirium generally comes on; the
tongue is smooth, exceedingly dry, and after
a while becomes livid; the respiration is
short and laborious; the eyes, which are
more prominent than in the acute plague,
are very red and full of ferocity; the face and
neck are turgid, at first red and afterwards
livid; vomiting seldom comes on spontane-

(κ) This anxiety about the præcordia may be regarded
as a pathognomonic symptom of the plague in its most
acute type. It is so excessive that the patients are at a loss
for words capable of expressing it. It does not consist in
a violent pain, but in a certain oppressive, suffocating, and
altogether intolerable sensation at the pit of the stomach.
In this state, they make known their anguish and show
the danger they are in by sighs, tears, and lamentations,
writhing their bodies in the most violent manner, and,
especially when their delirum comes on, falling down
upon the ground or floor, and crawling about as long as
any muscular power remains. Others who are affected
with extreme debility from the first, although they feel
the same anguish, are not capable of tossing and writhing
themselves about so much.

ously.

oufly. Such as are feized with thefe violent
fymptoms feldom live more that twenty-four
hours. Moft of them die apopledtic, or in
a ftate of convulfive fuffocation (L); fome,
however, expire in a more placid manner.
After death the bodies turn livid in thofe
parts where nature had endeavoured to throw
out buboes; and dark-coloured fpots and vibices appear in different places. In the other
mode of attack, the patients are affected with
debility from the beginning, which, together with the anxietas præcordiorum, increafes every moment; fo that unlefs timely
relief be given, death fpeedily comes on.
In thefe cafes, the pulfe is very quick, but
fmall, feeble, and at length imperceptible.
Sometimes there is a low delirium; but in
many inftances the patients are fenfible to
the laft. Thefe are all the febrile fymptoms
that are obfervable. Rudiments or germs of
buboes are feen upon the dead bodies.

(L) In the fame manner as thofe who die of the catar-
rhus fuffocativus.

Of

Of thefe two varieties of the plague in its moft acute form, the firft was obferved to take place in perfons of a robuft conftitution and in full health, after making too hearty a meal on food not eafily digefted, or eating too much fruit, &c. The other variety attacked thofe who were under the influence of terror, or after immoderate venery, bleeding, &c.

The very acute type of the plague is lefs frequent than the other types, and often deftroys the patient before medical affiftance is called in; in fo much that he who appeared well yefterday, is to day carried to his grave. In this fpecies of the plague, I never faw perfect carbuncles and exanthemata; but buboes come out quickly after the attack, and are feen confiderably elevated and livid in the dead bodies.

Such is the defcription of fymptoms given by *Orræus*, a diligent and accurate obferver. That publifhed by *Samoïlowitz* *,

* Memoire fur la Pefte, qui en 1771, ravagea l'Empire de Ruffie, fur tout Mofcou, &c. par M. D. Samoïlowitz. A Paris, 1783.

although

although it is not fo circumftantial nor fo well digefted, coincides in all effential points with the above. This laft author confiders the plague under three different afpects or varieties, which correfpond to the *three periods of its beginning, its height, and its decline.* In the firft and laft period, carbuncles and confluent petechiæ, or broad maculæ, are very rarely met with; whereas in the middle period, when the diforder rages with the greateft fury, they both occur in one and the fame fubject, and denote the utmoft danger. At this period, (viz. when the plague is at its height) the peftilential particles being more virulent, more volatile, and more fubtile, enter the body more readily, act upon it with greater force, and produce a difeafe which runs its courfe with greater rapidity than in either of the other two degrees or varieties of the plague.

The fymptoms in *the firft period of the plague* are few and moderate; they are for the moft part reducible to head-ache, vomiting,

ing, and buboes; petechiæ rarely appear *, or if they do, they are diftinct and very fmall; carbuncles are hardly ever feen. This degree of the plague terminates favourably by a fuppuration of the buboes, often without any affiftance from art. It may therefore be termed the mild or benignant form of the plague.

The *next degree or variety* is that which occurs when the plague is at its height. This is the moft terrible form of the diforder. All the fymptoms are marked with violence. The head-ache is inceffant, and the vomiting recurs frequently; the external characters are numerous; carbuncles appear in various parts of the body; the petechiæ or maculæ are very large and confluent, and often turn to carbuncles a fhort time before death. This happens in the following manner: two,

* This remark refpecting the rare occurrence of petechiæ in the beginning of the plague is contrary to the obfervations of *Mertens* and *Orræus*. Mr. *Samoïlowitz* did not fee much of the plague at Mofcow in the beginning; he was chiefly employed in the care of the peft-hofpitals during the height of the diforder. Tr.

three,

three, or four large petechiæ run together
and form a yellow pustule; sometimes a similar pustule rises upon each petechia; in
either case, on opening the pustules, a true
carbuncle appears beneath. In some instances the patient is seized from the first
with a furious delirium; at other times this
delirium or phrenitic state does not supervene
until the second, third, or fourth day. If
this disorder of the brain continues until the
seventh day, there are hopes of recovery; on
the other hand, if the delirium ceases on or
after the first or second day, and the patient
becomes tranquil and feeble, such an alteration is a certain presage of death. If this
change took place in the morning, the patients
died in the evening; if in the evening, they
did not live over the night. At other times
torpor came on, and continued through the
whole of the disease, so that the patients
died without pain, or at least without ap-
pearing to suffer any. In some instances, on
being asked how they were, the patients replied, " very well," and called for meat and
drink; but soon after they sunk into a de-
liquium

liquium animi, in which they remained motionless, and died.—The pulse was irregular from the beginning. When there was violent head-ache, with high delirium, &c. the pulse was full, hard, ſtrong, and quick; on the other hand, when theſe ſymptoms ceaſed, whether ſhortly after the attack or after the ſecond or third day, the pulſe then became ſoft, feeble, intermitting, and not to be felt *. In many inſtances the ſkin was dry and hot, and the patients complained of a burning ſenſation, both outwardly and in-

---

* Feeling the pulſe of impeſted patients with the bare fingers, is always attended with great riſk of taking the contagion, which is ſo readily communicated by contaꞔt. This, however, did not deter Mr. *Samoïlowitz*, from feeling the pulſe in all the different forms or varieties of the plague, in the uſual manner; though others took the precaution of putting on gloves, or having a leaf of tobacco applied to the patient's wriſt before they ventured upon this examination. It is evident that much reliance cannot be placed upon the reports of thoſe who felt the pulſe through the intervening ſubſtances juſt mentioned. This and other obſervers have remarked, that after the pulſe was once aſcertained in each form or variety of the plague, it became unneceſſary to feel it any more. According as the head-ache was either dull or acute, the delirium high or low, &c. the phyſician could pronounce, without feeling the wriſt, upon the ſtate of the pulſe. Tr.

wardly;

wardly; in others the heat was not fo great; in fome the fkin was yellow; in others it had a pale corpfe-like appearance, joined with great flabbinefs. The diarrhœa was often accompanied with an incontinence of urine, both which it was fometimes impoffible to check; in fuch cafes, thefe fymptoms (occurring together) were the fore-runners of death. The diarrhœa was common to both fexes; but the incontinence of urine was obferved in female patients only.

3. *The third degree or variety of the plague* occurred in the decline of the epidemic. Its fymptoms are the fame as thofe which take place in the firft type; and, therefore, to avoid repetition, we refer to that *.

B. *Quef-*

* If the fymptoms in the decline of the plague were precifely the fame with thofe in the beginning, there would be but two types or varieties of the diforder; the 1ft, comprehending the phenomena of the plague at its beginning and in its decline; and the 2d, the phenomena which belong to its height. But from the obfervations of *Mertens* and others, it appears that although there is a great refemblance between the plague at its decline and in the begin-

B.

Queftions relative to the Nature, Prevention and curative Treatment of the Plague.

The queftions propofed by Prince *Orlow* to the phyficians, and furgeons, were

1. In what manner is the contagion, which is making fuch great ravages in this place, propagated?

2. What are the fymptoms which fhow that a perfon is infected with this diforder? In what refpects does it differ from other malignant fevers, and what fymptoms has it in common with them? How is the patient

beginning (viz. that in both cafes the fymptoms are lefs violent and lefs fatal than thofe which occur in the middle period or at the height of the epidemic) yet there is alfo a difference between them, the plague in the beginning of its career being accompanied with petechiæ and other fpots, as well as buboes; whereas at the decline, fcarcely any other external marks, befides buboes, are obferved. Tr.

himfelf

himself to know that he is attacked with this dreadful diforder, fo as to be able to apply for help at the very beginning? How are thofe who are conftantly with the fick, to know the diforder, fo as to be put upon their guard againft taking infection? And, laftly, how is the phyfician to be certain that it is the difeafe in queftion *, in order that all poffible means may be immediately employed to fave the life of the patient?

3. Each of you is required to defcribe accurately the fymptoms of this diforder through its whole courfe and under all its forms, noticing in what order the fymptoms fucceed each other, more efpecially what the fymptoms are which accompany each crifis, and what thofe are which denote more or lefs danger: laftly, in what fpace of time, in what manner, and with what outward marks this contagious diforder terminates, whether it be in recovery or in death?

* We fuppofe this query to relate to thofe phyficians who received reports from the furgeons and their affiftants, without vifiting the fick themfelves. Tr.

4. What

4. What are the medicines which have hitherto been adminiſtered in the different caſes, in what doſes, in what ſtage of the diſorder, and with what ſucceſs? The general reſult of theſe obſervations will determine which is the eaſieſt and moſt ſucceſsful method of cure.

5. What is it neceſſary for the patient to obſerve when he is taking the remedies, and when he is not; and what ſort of regimen is beſt ſuited to promote the cure?

6. Laſtly, each of you is required to make known, according to his own judgment and experience, what appear to be the beſt and ſureſt methods by which individuals may eſcape this terrible ſcourge, and by which it may be checked, and if poſſible entirely eradicated; but theſe methods muſt be ſimple and eaſily put in practice.

My anſwers to theſe queſtions were as follow:

1. That

1. That this contagious diforder was propagated by touching the fick or dead bodies; by handling infected goods, fuch as clothes, furniture, and the like; by the patient's breath; or by the air of a room, confined and loaded with effluvia from the bodies of the fick; but not at all by the common atmofphere *. Hence thofe who avoid all communication with the fick, and never meddle with infected things, remain free from the plague, although they live in the fame territory or in the fame town where it is making its ravages; whilft the poor, not fhunning communication with the fick, and putting on infected clothes, which they buy cheap or get by inheritance, are continually expofed to the contagion, and are confequently thofe who are chiefly attacked by

---

* Although Dr. *Mertens* maintains (what we believe no phyfician in thefe days will be difpofed to contradict) that the contagion is not diffeminated by the common atmofphere; yet, in other parts of his Treatife, he admits that the air may become infected to a certain diftance by a great number of bodies, dead of the plague, lying unburied. Tr.

F

the

the plague *. Now, if the caufe of the plague exifted in the atmofphere, or that it was carried by it in a ftate of activity from one place to another, it fhould follow, that all the inhabitants of the fame territory, or at leaft of the fame town, rich as well as poor, fhould be equally attacked by it; but

* There are many reafons why the poor muft be the the chief victims of the plague, whenever it rages in any country ; for 1ft, They are the perfons who are employed to remove or deftroy infected goods, to carry away and bury the dead, &c. 2dly, As they live in fmall, crouded habitations, when any one of them is attacked by the dif- order, all the reft of the fame family are expofed to the contagion, in confequence of breathing an air tainted by the breath and other effluvia of the fick. 3dly, They are generally deftitute of nurfes and other neceffary attendants, and particularly they cannot have that change of linen, which contributes in a very great degree to carry off the contagion and promote the recovery. 4thly, When the plague is at its height, the number of fick is fo great that it becomes impoffible for the phyficians and furgeons to vifit all of them, even once in twenty-four hours, though to be of real fervice, the vifits fhould be repeated, in every family, twice within that fpace of time. Laftly, They have not wherewithal to procure themfelves the proper food and diet ; or, if thefe are provided for them out of the parochial funds, by the contributions of the wealthy, or by government, they do not ftrictly adhere to them, but fly to fpirituous liquors and other hurful things. Tr.

this

this is not the cafe. All, therefore, that can be attributed to the atmofphere, with regard to the plague, is, that according to its diffe-rent temperature, it difpofes the human body more or lefs to receive the contagion; and that according as its temperature is greater or lefs, it renders the peftilential miafm more or lefs violent, or even deftroys it; which, indeed, feems to have been the opinion of other writers on this fubject*. We have feen in the preceding narrative, that the cold of winter blunted, and as it were froze the pef-tilential virus, whilft the heat of fummer rendered it more active and volatile; never-thelefs, at both thefe feafons, the atmofphere was as healthy as ufual.

2. That it was fometimes difficult to af-certain the exiftence of the plague on its firft appearance; but that afterwards it was at-

* *Sydenham* Oper. Sect. II. Cap. 2. and *Van Swieten* Comment. Tom. V. § 1407.

We have deemed it fufficient to refer to thefe authors, without tranfcribing the paffages which Dr. *Mertens* has introduced. Tr.

tended

tended by certain marks, which diſtinguiſh
it from every other diſeaſe. Theſe charac-
teriſtic marks are petechiæ, buboes, and carbuncles. When theſe occur in a diſorder
which is very rapid in its progreſs, is accompanied with fever (unleſs when it deſtroys
ſuddenly) and is highly contagious, there can
be no doubt that ſuch a diſorder is the
plague *.

To determine with certainty whether a diſorder which prevails in any place is the
plague, it muſt have all the ſymptoms which
I have juſt deſcribed in one or more patients.
Theſe ſymptoms taken ſingly, do not con-
ſtitute the plague; for many other diſor-
ders are equally rapid in their courſe; petechiæ appear in common putrid fevers; in
ſome malignant fevers carbuncles are met

* The author includes in his definition of the plague
the circumſtance of the diſorder being brought by infeƈted
perſons or goods from Egypt, or ſome other province of the
Turkiſh empire; but as this is a circumſtance which relates merely to its origin, without ſerving to mark its pro-
perties or pourtray its features, we thought it foreign to a
definition, and have accordingly omitted it. Tr.

with;

with; buboes are produced by the venereal
diſeaſe and ſcurvy; and ſome times, though
very rarely, a criſis happens in putrid fevers
by abſceſſes forming under the arm-pits; but
theſe abſceſſes ariſe later in theſe caſes than
they do in the plague, and moreover they are
not accompanied with buboes and the other
ſymptoms which characterize the plague.
The high degree of contagion by which the
diſorder is propagated from one perſon to
another, enters neceſſarily into the definition
of the plague; without it there is no plague.
In a word, if there is a frequent communication, either by commerce or in conſequence
of war, with Turkey or Egypt, and ſome
perſons, or a great number of perſons, are
attacked with a diſorder which correſponds
exactly to the definition above given, it is
certain that it is the plague.

3. For the anſwer to this third queſtion,
the reader has only to revert to the deſcrip-
tion of ſymptoms in note A of the Addenda. As for the prognoſis, it is attended
with great uncertainty in caſes of the plague.

In

In some inftances, an indifpofition apparently
flight, is quickly followed by death; whilft
others who feem to be on the point of death,
recover *. In general, when the buboes
fuppurate well, and there is a feparation of
the efchars from the carbuncles, accompanied with an abatement of the other fymptoms, a favourable prognoftic may be given.

4. That hitherto medicine had done very
little good, the diforder being fo rapid in
its courfe as not to allow time for the remedies to act; but that the Peruvian bark and
mineral acids, in large dofes, ought, in my
opinion, to form the bafis of the curative
treatment.

From the preceding hiftory of the plague
it appears, that thofe who are attacked with
this diforder are affected with nervous fymptoms before the fever comes on, and that the
fever itfelf is of a highly putrid nature, ac-

* See *Chenat* de Pefte, p. 93, and *Ruffell's* Aleppo,
p. 229 and 235.

companied

companied with marks peculiar to itſelf, and
which diſtinguiſh it from all other fevers.
The proportion of thoſe in whom the plague
appears under the form of an inflammatory
fever, is very ſmall: and this happens only
in the beginning of the diſorder, in plethoric ſubjects; and that in theſe inſtances,
from being inflammatory it quickly becomes
putrid. Thus there are two ſets of ſymptoms in the plague, viz. thoſe which depend
on nervous irritation, and thoſe which depend on the putrid condition of the blood.
The firſt I call the *nervous*, and the ſecond
the *putrid ſtate.*

In the firſt, or nervous ſtate, the indica-
tion is to promote perſpiration by warm aci-
dulated drinks, ſuch as infuſions of tea and
other herbs mixed with lemon juice or vinegar, camphorated emulſions, camphor julep
with vinegar and muſk, &c. If ever bleeding is proper, it is at this period, and in plethoric ſubjects.

In

In the second, or putrid state, vomits, the Peruvian-bark, and mineral acids are the most promising remedies. The violence and rapidity with which the difeafe runs its courfe, require that thefe medicines fhould be adminiftered in powerful dofes. In the month of September, a woman, aged twenty-four, was feized with head-ache, fever, and vomiting; fhortly after, a bubo came out on the right groin, and another under the arm-pit on the fame fide, of the fize of a hazel nut; the next day fmall petechiæ appeared over the whole body; fhe was weak and drowfy; the tongue was white and moift; the urine pale; and fhe complained of head-ache and oppreffion about the præcordia. After I had made her vomit by giving her twenty grains of ipecacuanha, I ordered her a very ftrong decoction of Peruvian bark, to a quart of which were added a drachm and a half of the extract of the fame bark, a drachm of the acid elixir of vitriol of the London Pharmacopœia, and an ounce of fyrup of marfhmallow; fhe took three ounces of this mixture every other hour, and befides this, fhe alfo took

four

four times in the day, half a drachm of
Peruvian bark in powder. For her common
drink, she had a decoction of barley, acidu-
lated with spirit of vitriol. The buboes
increased gradually, insomuch that in the
space of a few days they were as large as
walnuts; they continued in this state, without any signs of suppuration. The patient
began to mend regularly, and at the end of
a week, she was almost entirely recovered;
she was then removed, in spite of all my re-
monstrances to the contrary, to the hospital,
from which she was dismissed a short time
afterwards, and came to see me, in perfect
health.

By this mode of treatment I am persuaded
that those who have the plague in its moderate
and flow form, may be rescued from death.
This is further confirmed by the cases of three
children, one of whom was only a year old,
and the two others still younger; each of
them had a pestilential bubo in the groin,
accompanied with fever and great debility.
After they had taken the decoction of Peru-

vian

vian bark, mixed with the extract, they got
better; the buboes ripened and yielded a
good pus. Two of these children got quite
well; the third was carried off during his
convalescence, by convulsions occasioned by
the teeth. Although this happened in the
month of December, when the disorder, being more mild, allowed many to recover;
nevertheless these facts serve to establish the
efficacy of the remedy, since the symptoms
of the plague are always worse in children
than adults, and its good effects were seen
in all the three patients at the same time.

But the cure of the plague by the mineral
acids and Peruvian bark, is only to be expected when the disease appears under its less
violent forms. In a great number of instances (where the disease has been more violent) these remedies have been prescribed, not
only without effecting a cure, but even without retarding death for a moment. Various
other medicines, such as theriaca (which has
been so improperly cried up in the plague)
camphor, dulcified spirit of nitre, &c. have in
like

like manner failed ; fo that we are compelled
to acknowledge, that the plague (under its
more violent forms) is of fuch a malignant
nature as not to yield to any medicines with
which we are yet acquainted, howfoever well
adapted they may, *à priori*, feem to be for
getting the better of this diforder. From
analogy and the preceding facts, I am inclined
to place more reliance upon the Peruvian
bark and acids, given in large dofes, than upon
any other remedy ; joining with them, to
obviate debility, camphor, elixir of vitriol,
wine, and blifters. Some were relieved by
gentle emetics, fuch as ipecacuanha. A
furgeon who had brought with him from
England a great quantity of *James's* Powder,
prefcribed it to feveral patients ; but I never
heard that it anfwered better than ipecacuanha
or other emetics *. Purgatives, even of the
moft

---

* From the manner in which the author makes mention of *James's* powder, it appears that it was adminiftered
in fuch large dofes as produced vomiting. It fhould have
been given in fmall quantities, fo as to have acted as a dia-
phoretic

moſt gentle ſort, were hurtful; they brought
on a diarrhœa which it was ſcarcely poſſible
to check, and which weakened the patients
exceedingly. I conſider bleeding to be very
improper in the plague; nevertheleſs I
would not forbid it entirely, where the diſeaſe, in plethoric ſubjects, aſſumes an inflammatory form, and is accompanied with phre-
nitis; which, however, was ſeldom the caſe
in the plague at Moſcow *.

5. That during the convaleſcence, wine,
malt-liquor, kuas (the ſmall beer of Ruſſia)

phoretic, both alone, and in conjunction with opiates.
Perhaps, however, it may be objected that this and other
antimonials, in ſmall doſes, repeated at intervals of three or
four hours, are too tardy in their operation for a diſeaſe ſo
rapid in its progreſs? In larger doſes they would be apt to
purge. Thus there ſeems to be little encouragement for
adminiſtering them in any way, in caſes of the plague.
Tr.

* As the author's obſervations relative to the treatment of the buboes and carbuncles, coincide with thoſe
of other writers on this ſubject, they have been pur-
poſely omitted. See *Ruſſell* on the Plague, Book II.
Chap. V. Tr.

light

light vegetable food *, and above all fresh air, were proper and necessary: The same diet which is suited to putrid fevers is equally suited to the plague. Nothing answers better for raising the drooping spirits and recruiting the strength of the weak and convalescent, than well fermented malt liquor, or wine and water.

6. That as to checking its progress and entirely eradicating the pestilence, that, in the present extended state of the disorder, would be attended with much difficulty; but that whatever tended to lessen the communication between the sick and healthy, and to prevent the latter from coming in contact with infected clothes, furniture, &c. would contribute to this end; and that I hoped the frost would not only weaken the contagion, but in a great measure destroy it.

---

* Why no animal food? *Orræus* found broths and soups seasoned with salt and vinegar, and having the fat taken off them, and even boiled meat of a light texture, to be very restorative to the convalescent. Tr.

When

When physicians of science and probity declare that they are convinced of the existence of the plague in any place, it is incumbent on the magistrates, without paying any regard to the contrary opinions of other practitioners, to take the necessary precautions for preserving the health of the public, by removing, as soon as possible, all infected persons, as well as those who are under suspicion of being infected, out of the town, to a house standing by itself, and to surround the building with guards, in order to cut off all communication. As it is of great importance in the beginning of the plague to suppress it in secret, an infected family may be removed in the night-time, without giving rise to any suspicions concerning the disorder; which if it has, as yet, appeared only in this family, may be thus extinguished, without exciting a general alarm *. But when

* If there should be any doubts respecting the nature of the disorder on its first appearance, and because, as yet, only a single family happens to be attacked with it; Dr. *Mertens* proposes that criminals condemned to death should be

when feveral families have become infected,
it is then no longer poffible to keep it a fecret
from the public, fince the precautions which
it is neceffary to employ muft make it
known. In fuch a cafe, the impefted, as
well as all thofe who have dwelt under the
fame roofs with them, muft be cut off from
all further communication with the reft of
the inhabitants. The clothes and furniture
belonging to the fick (excepting fuch things
as are of a hard and folid texture, which it
will be fufficient to wafh with vinegar) muft
be burnt. The goods that are thrown into
the fire muft not be touched with the hands,
but be taken hold of by tongs and poles fur-

be fhut up with the fick, and be made to wear their clothes.
Thus in two or three weeks, according as they became
infected or not, it would be decided whether the diforder
was the plague. But in a free country, like England,
neither the removing of a family in the night-time, under
the circumftances juft mentioned, nor the expofing of criminals to the contagion, are meafures which would be
deemed juftifiable. Indeed, it feems almoft impoffible to
ftifle the plague, in any country, in the very beginning,
before it has become publicly known and excited a general
alarm. Tr.

nifhed

nifhed with hooks at the end *; in the fame
way, the dead bodies are to be put into the
carts, that carry them to the burying-
grounds. Perfons who may be relied on,
fhould be appointed to fee that all thefe directions are ftrictly complied with. The
relations and friends of the fick fhould be
perfuaded to burn the clothes and other effects which they may at different times have
received; and the health of fuch friends and
relatives fhould be well watched by the phyficians.

A Board of Health, compofed of fome
perfons of rank, two or three phyficians,
and as many of the principal citizens, fhould
regulate, under the authority of the magif-
trates. all matters relative to the health and

* Thofe who are employed to burn the goods, fhould
not ftand too near the fire, fo as to be expofed to the thick
fmoke which arifes from it; and the more effectually to
deftroy the peftilential particles, it may be ufeful to throw
fome gun-powder or nitre into the fire. It is infinitely
better to burn the infected goods than to bury them, as
fome authors recommend; fince people may be tempted
by avarice to dig them up again.

safety

fafety of the inhabitants. This Board or Committee fhould divide the town into quarters or diftricts, in each of which they fhould appoint a phyfician to vifit the fick; they fhould enjoin the inhabitants to apprize them whenever any individual in a family is taken ill; and they fhould order that no perfon be buried until the corpfe fhall have been examined by one of the faculty, and a note be given certifying the diforder of which the perfon died. If there fhould not be a fufficient number of phyficians, the furgeons may be employed in this bufinefs.

The poverty of the common people, and the avarice of others in better circumftances, have, in all places and at all times, been the chief caufes by which the contagion has been propagated. The poor man, who dreads hunger more than death, cannot bear to fee himfelf deprived of the pittance of property left him by a relation or friend, and accordingly endeavours to fecure in fecret all that he can; whilft the avaricious man, delighted

with

with the thoughts of making a good bargain,
buys what is offered for fale, regardlefs of
the rifk. he runs of taking the contagion.
There is but one effectual remedy for this
evil, which, as long as it fubfifts, renders
all precautions whatever of no avail. The
remedy I mean is to allow a fum of money
from the public treafury for the payment of
the value of the goods which are burnt. In
fact, the condition of thofe whofe family is
attacked with the plague is woful enough;
deprived of their friends and cut off from all
fociety, they have little elfe to expect but
death: is it fit, then, that their fituation fhould
be rendered ftill more deplorable by having
their goods taken from them and deftroyed,
without any compenfation; and thus to have
no other profpect left them but that of
extreme indigence, in cafe of recovery? Let
perfons be appointed to appraife fairly the
goods which are burnt, and pay for them accordingly; or, let the money be depofited in
the hands of fome banker, or of a committee chofen for that purpofe, with the claim-
ant's name, in order that if he recovers,

it

it may be given to him, or in cafe of death, to his heirs. Not only thofe among the poor who are ill of the plague, but thofe alfo who are fufpected of having the contagion, fhould be fed and maintained at the public expence; humanity, as well as the fafety of the reft of the inhabitants, requires that this fhould be done. A fufficiently large fum fhould be appropriated to this purpofe, in order that, in cafe of urgency, there may be no difficulties on this head. If every thing is arranged in this manner from the firft appearance of the plague, the expences will not be very heavy, the contagion will be eafily ftopped, and the evil will be ftifled in its infancy. When the diforder has ceafed, all who have recovered from it, as well as thofe who have attended upon the fick, fhould remain fhut up for fome time until all doubts are removed as to their being capable of communicating the contagion, on mixing with the inhabitants again. Forty days (whence the term *quarantine*) are the ufual probation; but although this fpace of time may be requifite for the complete purification of goods, it

feems

feems to be much longer than is neceffary in the cafe of infected perfons, or perfons merely fufpected of having the contagion *. Before thofe who have been performing quarantine are allowed to have communication with the reft of the inhabitants, they fhould be wafhed all over with vinegar, fhould put on new clothes (their old ones having been previoufly burnt, as well as their furniture, &c.) and have their houfes well fumigated. Befides all this, it will further be proper to make a ftrict fearch for feveral months after, in order to be fatisfied that the contagion is not concealed in any part of the town, and that nobody has locked up infected clothes or goods in chefts, trunks, &c. or hidden them in any other places; for the plague might, when leaft apprehended, fpring up again from fuch a fource. The peftilential germ confined in clothes or bales of merchandife acquires a greater degree of virulence, and may in that manner be tranfported to very great diftances, and be preferved for a great

* See *Chenot* de Pefte, p. 208.

length

length of time. The deadly power of this
poifon is fo much increafed by being fhut up
in bales of goods clofely packed and well
defended from the air, that there are inftances of perfons who were feized with the
moft violent fymptoms and fuddenly killed,
on opening them *. In the laft century, a
twelvemonth after the plague had ceafed at
Warfaw, *Erndtel*, who relates the following
anecdote, paffed through that town in order
to attend the Court to Marienburgh and
Dantzic : in the town of Langenfurt, a
coachman's wife, being near the time of
her lying-in, brought with her in the month
of October a mattrefs on which fome perfons,
who had died of the plague a year before,
had lain. Having made ufe of it, fhe was
foon feized with the fame diforder, accompanied with inguinal buboes, and was fhortly
afterwards delivered; but an hæmorrhage
from the womb coming on, fhe died, as well
as the child. The hufband, alfo, died foon

* *Antrechaux*, Relation de la Pefte, p. 65. *Chenot*,
de Pefte, p. 166.

after,

after, having buboes and carbuncles; and many other persons caught the infection, which proved fatal to more than twenty of them. This contagion continued to manifest itself until the month of February, without, however, occasioning any more deaths, the persons belonging to the Court being dispersed in different villages and country seats. It ceased altogether in the beginning of March *. After the plague has spread itself and become prevalent, its progress is resisted with much more difficulty, and it threatens to become a general calamity. We must not, however, wholly despair; for if, on the one hand, the Magistrates and the Committee of Health exert themselves to the utmost, and on the other, the inhabitants are tractable, the evil may yet be suppressed, especially if the season be favourable. The first object of attention is, to prevent it from being carried into the neighbourhood and other places. To this end, it will be proper to make known in a printed declaration, that

* *Erndtel* Warsavia physice illustrata, p. 171.

the

the disorder which rages is the plague; that the contagion does not exist in the air, and is only communicated by contact of the sick and infected goods: In this advertisement the inhabitants should be called upon to obey punctually the orders which may be given for the safety of the public at large, as well as of individuals; they should be warned against buying clothes or other effects which have been used; and dealers in second-hand goods and clothes should not be suffered to carry on their trade: Further, if the plague rages in one quarter of the town only, all communication between that part and the rest of the town should be immediately cut off.

In the beginning, when only a few families have become infected, the public safety requires that they should be sent out of the town, or at least removed to some detached building, so as to be deprived of all further intercourse with the rest of the inhabitants; but this should be done in a humane and soothing manner, and with as little inconvenience as possible to these unfortunate persons.

G 4　　　　　When

When the calamity, however, has arrived at such a pitch, that great numbers are attacked with the diforder, and that it has fpread itfelf over every part of the town; we can no longer hope to eradicate it entirely by thefe precautions. At this period it would be cruel and unfeeling to add to the fufferings of fo many afflicted families, by forcing away the fick from the healthy, by depriving the father of the prefence of his children, the wife of the attentions of her hufband, and the old man of the comfort of his family. Under fuch circumftances, we fhould only aggravate the evil, by compelling the fick to conceal their illnefs. Befides, it is impoffible to find buildings fufficiently large and convenient for fuch a vaft number of patients. Neverthelefs, every exertion muft be made to ftop the progrefs of this terrible diforder, which propagates itfelf by contagion, in every direction.

In this melancholy fituation what adds to the diftrefs is, that it is difficult to contrive meafures which fhall on the one hand be con-

fiftent

fiftent with the humanity with which the unfortunate fufferers fhould be treated, and on the other, with the public fafety. If you drag from their houfes the fathers of families, mothers, and children, and thruft them into hofpitals, you rob them of the only confolation which is left them, you heap mifery upon mifery, and plunge them into defpair, from which it is impoffible for them to recover. On the other hand, although the contrary plan may feem more humane, it is neverthelefs equally cruel and fatal to the public at large to neglect all precautions, and to let the contagion take its own courfe; for in that cafe many towns and whole provinces would become a prey to the peftilence. We muft, therefore, take the mid-way between thefe two extremes.

Let an hofpital with the houfes near it, or a whole fuburb *, be appropriated for the

recep-

---

* By being diftributed in this manner into feveral houfes the fick will be lefs hurtful to each other; they will breathe a purer air, and recover much fooner. *Mead* ad-

vifes

reception of the poor who are feized with
the plague; let every thing which is requifite for their fupport and cure be provided
there; and let them repair thither of their
own accord, and not be brought by com-
pulfion. Let other perfons be allowed to
remain with them, provided the infected
houfes have a common mark upon the doors,

vifes the impefted to be removed to tents pitched out of
the town. (This is not quite accurate. *Mead*'s words
are,—" as the advice I have been giving is founded
upon this principle, that the beft method for ftopping infection, is to feparate the healthy from the difeafed; fo in
fmall towns and villages, where it is practicable, if the
*found remove themfelves into barracks or the like airy habi-
tations*, it may probably be even more ufeful, *than to remove the fick*. This method has been found beneficial in
France after all others have failed.") Tr. I do not think
a better method for ftopping the contagion can be fug-
gefted; but the feafon of the year, climate, and other cir
cumftances muft often render this meafure impracticable;
in that cafe, the doors and windows of the fick-rooms
fhould remain open, and a free circulation of air be conftantly kept up. The expofure to the air and wind feems
to me to be the principal reafon why the plague makes lefs
havoc in armies that are encamped; for although the air
or wind has very little power over the poifon after it has
entered the circulation, neverthelefs it carries off the effluvia and diffipates them more quickly; fo that the found
are not fo readily infected by the fick.

by

by which they may be diftinguifhed from the reft, in order that found perfons who enter them may be put upon their guard. Let the Board of Health circulate printed directions how the uninfected are to manage when they approach the fick, warning them to keep the doors and windows open, to avoid the breath of the infected, and the effluvia from their bodies and excrements; to fprinkle the rooms frequently with vinegar; and to avoid, as much as poffible, touching with their bare hands either the bodies of the fick or infected goods; or if they have touched them, to wafh their hands immediately with vinegar.

Phyficians, furgeons, and nurfes, muft be appointed to take care of the impefted, and have handfome falaries allowed them *.

---

* The phyficians and furgeons, and all thofe who are about the fick, fhould put over their clothes a cloak made of oil-cloth; they fhould wear gloves and boots made of the fame material, which fhould be frequently wafhed with vinegar; and they fhould hold before the mouth and nofe, a fponge moiftened with vinegar. On other prefer-vatives, fee D.

The

The Magiſtrates ſhould take care that the dead bodies do not remain unburied longer than is abſolutely neceſſary for determining the diſeaſe by which life was deſtroyed.

Thoſe who are employed in burying the dead ſhould be protected from the contagion, by having cloaks and gloves of oil-cloth, which ſhould be frequently waſhed with vinegar; and that they may not touch the dead bodies with their hands, they ſhould be provided with hooks and other inſtruments for lifting them up.

The burying-grounds ſhould be out of the town, and at ſome diſtance from the highroads; the corpſes ſhould be thrown into deep trenches, and be immediately covered over with a thick layer of earth, not only to prevent the effluvia that would otherwiſe ariſe from them, but alſo to ſecure them from dogs and crows.

Although, as I have before remarked, the atmoſphere at Moſcow, even when the

plague

plague was at its height, was not at all vitiated, and by no means contagious, not only
in the winter but alſo in the middle of ſummer, when the heat is as great as in any other
parts of Europe, excepting ſuch as lie immediately to the ſouth; yet, if a great number of bodies dead of the plague are ſuffered
to lie unburied and putrefy, they may im-
pregnate the air with their effluvia to ſuch a
degree as to render the atmoſphere (otherwiſe incapable of propagating the contagion)
infectious, eſpecially in ſummer, and thereby
cauſe it to ſpread inevitable deſtruction to the
neighbourhood. It is well known that the
carcaſes of all animals in a ſtate of corruption,
fill the ſurrounding atmoſphere with effluvia
that are accompanied with an intolerable
ſtench, and that theſe effluvia, though they
do not produce the plague, are nevertheleſs
the cauſe of putrid, malignant fevers. Accounts are given by ſeveral authors of ſuch-
like epidemic diſeaſes being produced by the
fætor exhaled from the dead bodies left on the
field of battle, or from the bodies of animals
putrefying in ſtagnant waters or on the banks

of

of rivers. Among others, *Forestus*, (Lib. 4. Obf. ix. Tom. 1.) gives the hiftory of a very malignant epidemic, occafioned by an enormous fifh of the whale kind, which lay corrupting on the fea-fhore. But how much more pernicious effects muft the putrefaction of bodies dead of the plague have, fince in this diforder the fimple effluvia from the fick are fo fatal to perfons in health ?

(The obfervations which follow on the airing of goods, on quarantine, &c. coincide fo much with thofe that are to be found in every treatife on the plague, that they are omitted by the Tranflator.)

C.

Of the Antipeftilential Fumigating Powders.

The houfes and rooms of perfons infected with the plague are purified by firing gunpowder in them. At Mofcow we employed
with

with fuccefs a powder, called *antipeftilential,*
of which fulphur and nitre formed the bafis,
fome bran and other vegetable fubftances,
fuch as abrotanum, juniper-berries, &c. together with certain refins, were added; but
in my opinion thefe refins are totally ufelefs,
and only increafe the expence *. The acid
vapours

* The following is the compofition of thefe fumigating
powders, as publifhed by the Council of Health. (See *Orræus,* p. 136, 137.)

The ftrong antipeftilential powder confifted of juniper
tops (cut fmall,) guaiacum fhavings, juniper berries, bran,
of each 6 ℔, nitre 8 ℔, fulphur 6 ℔, myrrh 2 ℔.

The weaker antipeftilential powder confifted of the herb
abrotanum 6 ℔, juniper tops 4 ℔, juniper berries 3 ℔,
nitre 4 ℔, fulphur 2½ ℔, myrrh 1½ ℔.

The odoriferous antipeftilential powder confifted of cala-
mus aromaticus 3 ℔, frankincenfe 2 ℔, amber 1 ℔, ftorax
and dried rofes, of each ½ ℔, myrrh 1 ℔, nitre 1 ℔ 8 oz.
fulphur 4 oz.

Of thefe powders, the firft was employed to fumigate
the houfes and goods of the infected, fuch as woollens,
furs, &c.; the fecond, for fumigating houfes only fufpected, and more delicate articles, which would have been
fpoiled by the firft; the laft was employed (by way of prevention) in inhabited houfes.

(We

vapours let loose on burning nitre and sulphur together, remain a long time suspended in the air *. The greater or less strength of these powders depends on the proportion of sulphur and nitre to the other ingredients. After burning the rags or other litter which may be found in the rooms, they are fumigated by throwing one of these powders on a chafing-dish or pan of coals, the doors and windows being shut, to keep in the smoke and vapour for a sufficient length of time. This vapour is hurtful to the lungs, and produces suffocation; hence the person who throws the powder upon the burning coals should get out of the room as fast as possible. This process is

(We are now acquainted with a mode of destroying contagion, much more simple and efficacious than that of fumigating with such compound and costly powders as those mentioned in the preceding note; we mean *the vapour extricated from nitre by means of the vitriolic acid.* See an Account of the experiments made on board the Union Hospital-ship, to determine the effect of the nitrous acid in destroying contagion. By James Carmichael Smith, M.D. &c. London, 1796. Tr.)

* The author adds, that the smoke from the vegetable substances burnt with them helps to keep the acid vapours longer suspended. We do not see how. Tr.

repeated

repeated three or four times in the space of
twenty-four hours for several days together;
after which the doors and windows are
thrown open.

D.

Of Preservative Remedies.

We shall content ourselves with abridging,
rather than translating at full length, what
the author offers on this head. Among other
preservatives, *issues* are taken notice of. The
author himself had one made in his left arm,
which he kept open for a twelvemonth; but
he is inclined to attribute his exemption from
infection rather to his having avoided the
contact of the sick and infected goods, than
to this remedy. It appears that four surgeons
at the principal pest-hospital died of the
plague, notwithstanding they had all of them
issues. Hence their preservative virtues may
be questioned; yet as they have been recommended by others, and are attended with
little inconvenience, he thinks it would be

H   proper

proper for thofe who are obliged to go among the infected, to have one made in the arm or leg, or both.—*Sweet spirit of nitre* was efteemed an excellent prefervative by fome; they took twenty or thirty drops of it upon a lump of fugar feveral times a day. Others took, with the fame intention, the *Peruvian bark* under different forms; but as they all kept out of the way of the contagion at the fame time, the prefervative powers of thefe remedies remain very doubtful. The common practice of carrying *camphor* in the pocket or fewed in the lining of the clothes, has nothing to recommend it. In like manner the *fmoking of tobacco*, though it has been fo ftrongly recommended by *Diemerbroeck* and others, is by no means a certain protection againft the contagion. The Turks, fays Dr. *Mertens*, are continually fmoking their pipes; and yet great numbers of them are fwept off by the plague every year. This reflection was not fufficient to do away the prejudice in its favour, fo difficult is it to deftroy a received opinion, howfoever falfe it may be. While the plague was raging at Mofcow, many Ruffian gentlemen and foreigners had

recourfe

recourse to the smoking of tobacco, as an in-
fallible prefervative. Those who were accuftomed to the pipe, fmoked oftener, whilft
others gradually brought themfelves to bear
it, until they faw fome among the foreigners
of the lower clafs carried off by the plague,
in fpite of the ufe of this remedy. The
mafter chimney-fweeper at the foundling-
hofpital, who had formerly ferved in the
Pruffian army, had fo much faith in the
fmoking of tobacco, that he was always feen
with a pipe in his mouth from morning to
night; and boafted that by this means he
fhould be proof againft the plague. Difre-
garding all other precautions, even when the
diforder was at its height, (viz. the month of
September) he got over the fences. in the
night-time, in order to go and fee his wife
and children who were in the town. He was
immediately feized with head-ach and vomiting, and the next day he had a bubo in the
groin and under the arm-pit, accompanied
with great debility and fever. He died at
the end of forty-eight hours. His apprentice,
twelve years of age, had a large flat bubo under
the armpit, and followed him foon after.

From

From the account publifhed by Count *Berchtold* at Vienna, in 1797, it would appear that the beft prefervative method is that recommended by Mr. *Baldwin*, the Britifh Conful at Alexandria. It confifts fimply in anointing the body all over with olive oil. According to the fame account, friction with warm oil is not only a prefervative, but alfo a curative remedy. See the fecond volume of *Duncan*'s Annals of Medicine.

E.

Of the means by which the Foundling-hofpital at Mofcow was kept free from the Plague

I fhall now give a particular account of the means by which the Foundling Hofpital was kept free from the plague, during the whole time that it raged at Mofcow; in the laft fix months of which it fwept off fo many thoufands of inhabitants. From this account it will eafily be feen how poffible it is in times of peftilence, to keep one's felf, one's family, and whole buildings, not only private but public, free from infection.

The

The Foundling Hofpital * is fituated in the middle of the city, at the conflux of the Yaufa and the Mofcua. It occupies a fpace of ground, at that time only inclofed by a hedge fix feet high, whofe circumference meafures nearly a French league. On this has been erected a building which might eafily be made to contain five thoufand foundlings. That part of it which was finifhed in 1769, contained one thoufand children and three hundred adults; the reft, confifting of maf-ters, fervants, workmen, and foldiers, who amounted to nearly one hundred, lived in houfes built of wood adjoining the ftone edifice and ftanding within the inclofure. This inclofure had three gates.

---

* This afylum of innocence and misfortune holds the firft place among all inftitutions of the fame kind in Europe. It was founded by the Emprefs Catherine the Second. Under the aufpices of this Sovereign, and by the great attention of Mr. *de Betzky*, to whom his country owes infinite obligations for the devotion of his time and fortune to the encouragement of the arts and the promotion of undertakings for the public good, this inftitution had nearly attained to perfection, at the time when this account of it was written.

In

In the month of July, as soon as I found
that the plague had spread itself in the town,
I requested the Governors of the hospital to
order all the gates to be shut, excepting that
where the porter lived; and not to suffer any
person to come in or go out, without permission from the principal inspector. I further
requested them to lay in a large stock, from
places not yet infected, of flour, cloth, linen,
shoes, and other necessaries. In the month
of August, when the plague was raging with
great fury, it was no longer permitted for any
one to enter but myself. Persons who lived
out of the enclosure were hired to purchase
all the necessaries of life, and to carry letters.
I gave the porter some written directions, in
which I put down every thing he was to allow to enter, and under what precautions.
The butcher threw the meat into large tubs
filled with vinegar, from which it was afterwards taken out by the under-cook. I prohibited the admission of furs, wool, feathers,
cotton, hemp, paper, linen, and silk; but I
allowed sugar-loaves to be received, after taking off the paper and packthread. Letters
were

were pricked through with a pin and afterwards dipped in vinegar, and dried in the
fmoke produced by burning juniper-wood.
The inhabitants of the building were allowed
to fpeak to their relations and friends, who
ftood at a certain diftance out of the gate *.
Being obliged to purchafe two hundred pair of
boots and fhoes, in the month of October;
I ordered them to be immerfed for fome
hours in vinegar, and afterwards dried.

I vifited all the fick in the houfe twice
every day; the found were examined by two
furgeons night and morning, who informed
me whenever they found any of them indifpofed. Whenever any fymptoms occurred
in a patient which appeared to me doubtful,
I kept fuch patient apart from the reft, until
I was fatisfied the diforder was not the
plague. In this manner I detected the plague

* I caufed to be fixed up at the gate near the porter's
lodge, two fets of railing, at the diftance of twelve feet
from each other. The people belonging to the hofpital
ftood at the inner railing, and thofe who came to fee them,
at the outer.

seven

feven times among the foldiers * and workmen belonging to the Foundling Hofpital;
but as I feparated them on the firſt appearance of the fymptoms, they none of them
infected the others, except the maſter chimney-fweeper, who gave it to his apprentice.
After the month of July, we ceafed to admit
any more foundlings or pregnant women. I
propofed to the Governors to hire, in the
mean while, a houfe for this purpofe in the
fuburbs, which was not determined upon
until the month of October †. At this time
there ſtill continued to die in the town above

---

* There was always a guard of twenty-two men and
an inferior officer. After July, I obtained an order not
to have them changed.

† It was not without great difficulty that we got a
houfe for quarantine, as well on account of obſtacles occafioned by the public calamity, as from the fcarcity of houſes
fufficiently roomy. Hence this bufinefs was not fettled
until October. In the mean time, many children continued to be expofed at the hofpital-gate. Some of thefe I
put into a wooden houfe in the vicinity ; and Mr. *de Durnowo* took others of them under his roof. As foon as the
above-mentioned quarantine-houfe was ready to receive
them, which was not the cafe till November, I fent them
thither.

a thoua thoufand perfons in a day. I had the children who were brought to this quarantine-houfe, ftripped to the fkin ; after which their clothes were burnt, their bodies wafhed all over with yinegar and water, and new clothes put upon them. I kept them for the fpace of a fortnight in three rooms detached from the reft; if, after that time, no figns of the plague appeared among them, they were put (having previoufly changed their clothes) each in the order in which he finifhed this firft term of probation, in the common dwelling-rooms of the quarantine-houfe; here they remained another fortnight, before they were removed to the Great Hofpital. I vifited every day thefe children and the lying-in women *. One infant was brought with a peftilential bubo, and two others, during the time of their quarantine, had the plague with buboes, as mentioned in a former part of this

---

* In this quarantine-houfe I alfo eftablifhed a fmall hofpital for the reception of pregnant women, and the care of them after their delivery, as long as the plague might continue. Mr. *de Durnowo* undertook the management of this eftablifhment.

I   treatife,

treatife. By putting them in feparate rooms along with their nurfes, the contagion was prevented from fpreading *. I had thus the happinefs of refcuing from death about one hundred and fifty children †, brought to the quarantine-houfe after the month of October. In the Spring of 1772, every thing was reftored to its former footing.

* As it was poffible for the plague, though it declined in the town, to have been kept up in this quarantine-houfe by the children that were daily brought there and by the lying-in women ; in order to provide againft fuch an event and in compliance with the orders of the Emprefs, Mr. *de Durnowo* and myfelf prefented a memoir, containing a detail of the regulations and precautions above-mentioned, to the Committee of Health, who were pleafed to fignify their approbation thereof.

(Here follows in the original, the letter of approbation from the Committee of Health, which though it is highly flattering to the author, is unimportant to the reader, and is therefore omitted by the Tranflator.)

† In the beginning of the year 1772, I had the remainder of the children who had been received into the quarantine-houfe, admitted, a few at a time, into the Great Hofpital. Their number, including orphans, whofe parents had been carried off by the plague, and new-born infants, amounted to one hundred and fifty.

THE END.

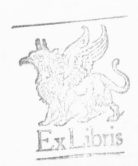